The Plant-based Powe

'This well-written, well-researched book makes it absolutely clear that a plant-based diet is best for your health, your body and your mind. Highly recommended!' Gene Stone, co-author of *How Not to Die*, author of 72 *Reasons to be Vegan*

'This book is brilliant. I've been involved in rugby as a player and coach at the highest level for over 22 years and this book provides real insight and evidence into how a plant-based nutritional programme can be a relevant and powerful alternative for athletes. In my experience there have been too many barriers and too much misinformation that hinder an athlete's nutritional choices and the viable options available. This book blasts through the confusion and provides a clear and pragmatic pathway to a healthy and robust plant-based lifestyle that will only enhance an individual's competitive performance. Every athlete, coach, trainer and medical practitioner in all sporting organizations should read this book and utilise the insights it offers' Les Kiss, Head Coach, London Irish Rugby Club

'TJ is a fantastic writer and authority on plant-based nutrition for athletes. *The Plant-based Power Plan* is packed with fresh knowledge, backed by the latest scientific research. Whether you're looking to kickstart a healthier lifestyle or take your training to the next level, this book has you covered' Plant-based Health Professionals UK

'An informative and interesting read regardless of whether you are an elite athlete or just want to improve physical endurance and overall wellbeing. I hold four Guinness World Records in marathon and ultra-running and have been vegan for almost five decades, and this book has really refreshed my attitude towards nutrition and brought many new perspectives and ideas to my plant-based lifestyle. I have taken on board many of its recommendations and suggestions for my own training and nutritional needs. A definite "must-read" for anyone interested, curious or already invested in plant-based living and thriving!' Fiona Oakes, four-time world-record-holding marathon runner

'If you want to know about plant-based living, this book sets that out very clearly: the why and the how, entirely based on science. It goes further than diet, reaching into issues of stress and sleep – this is a holistic lifestyle guide, from a scientist not a guru' Dale Vince, OBE, Chairperson, Forest Green Rovers FC, the world's first vegan football club

'Any athlete serious about their performance should consider a plant-based diet, and this book is brim full of the information you need to eat your way towards your full potential' Etienne Stott, MBE, London 2012 canoe slalom gold medallist

'*The Plant-based Power Plan* is a thoroughly researched and brilliantly informative guide, providing the fundamentals behind achieving optimal health and physical performance through the power and simplicity of plant-based foods. TJ shares valuable insight into his work helping elite sportspeople excel in their respective disciplines; offering tried-and-tested guidance for optimizing nutrition to enhance health and performance. TJ has done such an excellent job at breaking down stereotypes, providing evidence-based recommendations, and sharing simple and delicious plant-based recipes. This book is full of value for athletes and fitness enthusiasts alike, as well as anyone looking to improve their health through a plant-based diet' Ellie Woodhouse-Clarke, nutritional therapist and wellbeing expert

ABOUT THE AUTHOR

TJ Waterfall is a sports nutritionist specializing in plant-based nutrition. He works with elite vegan athletes, ranging from Premier League and international footballers, through Premiership rugby players, track and field athletes and endurance runners, to competitive weightlifters, boxers and swimmers. TJ is a registered nutritionist with the Association for Nutrition and has an MSc in Clinical and Public Health Nutrition from University College London, where he has worked in nutrition research. He writes for *Men's Fitness*, *Cycling Weekly* and *Outdoor Fitness*, among others, and speaks regularly at vegan festivals about the science-backed health benefits of plant-based diets. His website meatfreefitness.co.uk provides delicious vegan recipes, nutritional information, and fitness and lifestyle tips to help readers on their meat-free journey. He tweets @tjwaterfall and you can find him on Instagram @tj_waterfall.

The Plant-based Power Plan

Increase Strength, Boost Energy,
Perform at Your Best

TJ WATERFALL

PENGUIN LIFE

AN IMPRINT OF

PENGUIN BOOKS

PENGUIN LIFE

UK | USA | Canada | Ireland | Australia
India | New Zealand | South Africa

Penguin Life is part of the Penguin Random House group of companies
whose addresses can be found at global.penguinrandomhouse.com.

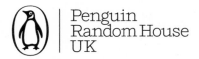

First published 2021
001

The information in this book has been compiled as general guidance on the specific subjects addressed.
It is not a substitute and not to be relied on for medical professional advice. Please consult your GP
before changing, stopping or starting any medical treatment or nutritional programme. So far as the
author is aware the information given is correct and up to date as at 4 November 2020. Practice,
laws and regulations all change and the reader should obtain up-to-date professional advice on any
such issues. The author and publishers disclaim, as far as the law allows, any liability arising
directly or indirectly from the use or misuse of the information contained in this book.

Text design by Couper Street Type Co.
Set in 13.5/16pt Garamond MT Std
Typeset by Jouve (UK), Milton Keynes
Printed and bound in Great Britain by Clays Ltd, Elcograf S.p.A.

The authorized representative in the EEA is Penguin Random House Ireland,
Morrison Chambers, 32 Nassau Street, Dublin D02 YH68

A CIP catalogue record for this book is available from the British Library

ISBN: 978–0–241–47244–6

www.greenpenguin.co.uk

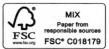

For Francesca and Isabella, who are my universe.

CONTENTS

CHAPTER 1

INTRODUCTION

One of the main questions I was asked when I first qualified and started practising as a plant-based nutritionist was: 'Can I *really* reach my health and fitness goals on a vegan diet?'

Times have changed. The benefits of adopting a vegan diet have been catapulted into the spotlight, even if not completely accurately, thanks to numerous documentaries and celebrities flying the plant-based-diet flag. The way we eat is changing, with studies showing that around half the UK are at least reducing the amount of meat they consume.

But for a lot of my clients and people I talk to, the biggest hurdle is knowing where to start themselves. It's about needing inspiration. It's about being provided with reassurance. It's about having the knowledge – and the confidence – that they're doing all they can to optimize their plant-based nutrition to help bring on their A-game.

And this is where the importance of evidence-based nutrition advice comes in. After I qualified with a first class master's degree in Clinical and Public Health Nutrition from University College London, I spent time working in public health nutrition with the NHS, I carried out further nutrition research at UCL, and I have gone on to train students and doctors in the health benefits of a plant-based diet and to work with world-class elite athletes to optimize their plant-based nutrition.

Because of my work in these fields, I've always required a very scientific mindset. This means having a constant thirst for knowledge, because the evidence is always evolving. When you think about it, nutrition is a relatively young science – compared to, say, physics or chemistry, which have been studied scientifically for centuries.

In nutrition, new studies often emerge that challenge current theories. Having a scientific approach means I can't be stuck in my ways (in contrast, some nutritionists base their entire career around a certain concept, and feel that changing their ways could jeopardize their reputation, even if new evidence suggests a more effective method, or that their current method could, even, be dangerous). I have to acknowledge change, and adapt my advice when needed. Scientists, by definition, always apply scepticism to any theory for this reason, because any concept should only be based on the **best available evidence** – which can change.

Most people are aware, at least to some degree, that what we eat can have profound effects on our health. But when it comes to performance, it often surprises me just how much people neglect their nutrition. Some athletes spend 20+ hours a week training, but invest very little time in learning about how best to use their diet to support recovery, and boost energy and power in training and competition. As you'll see throughout the book, the recovery from exercise, supported by your nutrition, is just as important – perhaps more important – than the training itself. If you're regularly spending several hours a week training, then taking the relatively short time to read this book and hone your nutrition could make all those hours much more productive and even more enjoyable, ultimately leading to huge progress in your sport or activity.

Having worked with plant-based elite sportspeople from a range of disciplines (premier league and international footballers, premiership rugby players, track and field athletes, endurance runners, competitive weightlifters, boxers), it's especially crucial to acknowledge any shortcomings in the evidence and tailor my advice accordingly, because the smallest of margins can make the difference between winning and losing. A discipline which perhaps exemplifies this the best is athletics, where tiny fractions of a second can separate first and second place. A top UK 100-metre sprinter recently asked me if a plant-based diet might help him out of a plateau he was experiencing – after working together closely to implement a nutrition plan he shaved two-tenths of a second off his personal best, which was enough to win his following three competition races. Using the scientific evidence, personalized to the athlete, is a powerful thing, and I'd like to help you in the same way, whatever your sport or activity may be.

This scientific approach couldn't be more pertinent when it comes to vegan nutrition. That's because for many people, including myself, the term 'veganism' – and what it represents – comes with a huge range of powerful emotions attached. For some, this could mean feeling opposed to veganism, because it contradicts their culture and traditions. Others may feel passionately about protecting animals and the environment. Either stance can distort how they interpret the evidence and the advice they give, knowingly or not.

For the purposes of transparency, it's worth mentioning that I fall into the category of people who care deeply about animal welfare and sustainability. But, in my experience, using the **scientific approach** and being honest about the considerations of any given diet is the best way to build trust and ultimately get the best results from my clients. Therefore, it's also the most helpful approach for advocating a healthy vegan diet, because one of the most effective ways to promote veganism is to help support people to thrive and lead by example.

Not only can a plant-based diet help your health and fitness flourish, but for me, vegan food is also a true celebration of flavour – I've always loved nothing more than creating bold, colourful dishes that celebrate the ingredients. Working in kitchens and teaching at a world-leading vegan cookery school has only brought out the 'foodie' in me further and made me realize the true variety and brilliance of a plant-based diet.

Think rich Indian curries, vibrant Mexican burritos, hearty French-style casseroles, spicy Chinese stir-fries . . . you can make too-good-to-be-true vegan versions of pretty much any cuisine from around the world. Seeing people's faces light up when they realize just how delicious and inventive plant-based food can be is another real highlight of my job.

Within the pages that follow, I will present you with:

- Trustworthy, evidence-based information to highlight the numerous health benefits of a well-planned vegan diet, which includes strong evidence showing a significant reduction in risk of developing the most prevalent chronic diseases.

- How to weigh up the evidence yourself, to help you cut through the noise and misinformation often represented in the media, so you can make the right decisions for yourself based on the best available evidence.

- Simple but comprehensive guidance to help make sure you're optimizing your plant-based nutrition, using scientifically proven nutritional advice to improve your energy and fitness while future-proofing your health.

- A breakdown of the key nutrients to consider as part of a healthy vegan diet (including vitamin B_{12}, vitamin D, omega-3, calcium and iodine), and the best sources for getting these into your diet.

- Evidence-based practical tips and guidance on how to surpass your sports and fitness goals, including tweaking your nutrition timing, maximizing muscle protein synthesis, getting the right energy balance, improving recovery times, and considering whether the use of ergogenic aids may be beneficial to you.

- Other proven essential lifestyle habits that will also have a huge impact on your health and fitness: sleep, movement, stress management and social connections.

- Advice on how to customize your own meal plan depending on your goals, including tips for those looking to gain or lose weight healthily and sustainably.

- A selection of 30 easy but tantalizingly tasty vegan recipes that also show you just how simple it is to incorporate all the key nutrients we cover naturally into your diet.

My goal with this book is to help you thrive on a plant-based diet. The evidence overwhelmingly suggests that it's one of the most effective ways to both improve long-term health and notice more immediate results in terms of energy, performance, and recovery. And in helping you to thrive on your plant-based journey, I hope you are filled with confidence to encourage and inspire those around you to consider giving it a try too. Because, ultimately, what's more important than your health, and the health of the ones you care about?

CHAPTER 2

WEIGHING UP
THE EVIDENCE

Have you ever spoken to someone who believes that the sugar in fruit is evil? They may have heard that it can make you overweight, promote inflammation, or cause diabetes. When I hear comments like this, my initial instinct, in all honesty, is to pull my hair out. When that urge subsides, though, I like to point out that all the science and data show that the exact opposite is true – in fact you'll see throughout this book how increasing consumption of whole plant foods, including fruit, helps achieve and maintain a healthy weight, reduce inflammation, protect against diabetes, and will help athletes take their performance to the next level.

This is just one of countless examples where the misinformation out there is so pervasive. At best, it can be misleading, or at worst, life-threatening. Many people I speak with base their nutrition habits on information they've gathered from social media, a quick Google search, or newspaper and magazine articles. Sometimes this works well, as there is *some* sound advice out there. But it's far outweighed by the seismic amount of misinformation, which makes things very confusing, even for health experts. It's all a bit of a minefield: there are conflicting messages, hidden agendas, and unqualified influencers all conspiring to confuse us!

That's why I feel it's so important to discuss how to weigh up the evidence before moving on to the following chapters. It serves two important purposes:

1. To highlight that the information provided throughout this book regarding plant-based diets is based on the best available research – not relying on research that's been 'cherry-picked' because it supports an argument. No evidence is perfect (as you will see), but I hope this will provide you with reassurance and confidence when planning your plant-based nutrition.

2. The world of nutrition is enormous, and while I hope this book covers the most important aspects you require for optimal health and fitness, there will inevitably be new questions that come up which you'd like answered. Therefore, this chapter will give you the tools you need to confidently research an unlimited number of further nutrition-related topics in the future.

This chapter will be particularly useful for anyone who's new to science and research. But even if you're well acquainted with research methods, I hope it'll get you thinking more about what you read. Throughout the book I point out some of the advantages and pitfalls of the evidence we cover, so gaining a good basic understanding here will be helpful in piecing together the evidence we discuss in later chapters too.

To get started, there are four questions I like to get my clients to really think about when doing their own research:

1.

Is this person qualified to talk about my nutrition?

This is particularly important because the word 'nutritionist' is not legally protected in the UK. That means anyone can technically call themselves a nutritionist, and give poor – or even dangerous – advice. And please remember, the number of followers they have on social media does not correlate with their level of expertise!

If you're looking for sound advice, it's essential to find a nutritionist who's appropriately qualified and preferably also registered with a trustworthy professional body. The largest professional body in the UK is the Association for Nutrition – this is the UK register of nutrition professionals, qualified in nutrition to at least degree level, who meet rigorous standards for scientifically sound, evidence-based nutrition, and its use in practice. Look for someone using the letters 'Nutr' after their name, which denotes their membership as a Registered Associate Nutritionist (ANutr) or if they also have several years of demonstrable experience then Registered Nutritionist (RNutr). Another protected body is the Sport and Exercise Nutrition Register (SENr), which is a similar voluntary register designed specifically for sport and exercise nutritionists. Being registered with both of these, I can attest that registration is not simple: it requires constructing a portfolio of qualifications, experience, research, and evidence of continuing professional development (CPD), such as attending seminars, courses and reading, to continually maintain, update and extend knowledge.

This is still not a guarantee that the information they provide is perfect, and you should always bear in mind the remaining three questions below. It also shouldn't rule out nutritionists qualified in other areas, including alternative therapies such as herbal medicine or kinesiology, as these approaches can unquestionably work for some people. However, if you're looking for advice that's based on the best science and research, then finding a Registered Nutritionist, qualified to at least degree level, is a good place to start.

Also remember that while medical doctors go through many years of training, unfortunately the current level of nutrition contained within their training is minimal – often a total of just 1–2 days. So, while doctors have an amazing amount of life-saving knowledge, they shouldn't necessarily be the first port of call for nutrition advice (unless they've voluntarily studied nutrition on top of their medical training).

2.

Does this sound too good to be true?

The promise of immediate improved health or enhanced performance can be incredibly alluring – it's a natural human desire to want good things to happen to us, and to want them fast. The culture of instant gratification in modern life means we've come to expect almost immediate results, even with our health, and we're often happy to part with considerable sums of money to achieve it. Unfortunately, there are many companies and individuals that are all too willing to take advantage of these desires and capitalize on the opportunity.

Well, when it comes to health and nutrition, there are no short cuts or miracle foods you can eat in isolation that will cure you of all your ailments. The truth is, the science of good nutrition is all about balance and variation – but this doesn't always sell products or make the headlines, which is why it's so underreported in the media. Of course, there are important changes you can make to your diet that will have a profound effect on your health, energy and performance, but these benefits aren't achieved through any miracle product or superfood alone (there's no regulated definition for 'superfood', but they generally offer particularly high levels of a desirable nutrient).

Don't get me wrong, some foods that have been given superfood status (such as kale, broccoli and blueberries) are highly nutritious and can be great to include in your diet. The reason alarm bells ring when I read promises of powerful foods with special abilities to promote weight loss or heal disease is because in these cases the term 'superfood' is clearly more useful for driving sales than for promoting optimal nutrition. In fact, the term 'superfood' alone often causes people to focus on just a few specific foods, blinding them to other equally nutritious options that aren't as hyped, which can lead to less variation in the diet and even a poorer overall diet quality.

Perhaps the advice you're reading advocates the use of a 'detox' product. Again, this is almost certainly sales-driven rather than science-based. Detoxification, by definition, refers to the removal of toxins from the body. If products are science-based, it should be possible to state which specific toxins are claimed to be removed, so you can objectively test whether there really is a detoxifying effect. As with superfoods, the promises of detoxing can lead to an overall decrease in diet quality – consumers often believe they can eat less healthily now (or even perhaps drink more alcohol or smoke) because they can simply 'detox' later. This just isn't how the body works.

3.

Are they presenting a balanced argument?

Looking at the best science and evidence when it comes to nutrition often doesn't result in clear-cut answers. For most topics there are exceptions, nuances and as-yet-unknowns, and therefore arguments for both sides of pretty much any debate. The truth is, especially when it comes to sports nutrition, that the right answers should usually depend on the individual's circumstances. That's why it's so difficult to simplify and condense complex nutrition research, accounting for all the nuances and individual variation, into an infographic or the small number of characters allowed in a social media post. Any article that intensely argues one side of a topic without consideration to the counterarguments is a warning sign to me that the writer:

- Hasn't researched the topic thoroughly.
- Is trying to sell me something.
- Doesn't understand that our bodies, circumstances and goals are incredibly individual and have unique needs.
- May have a hidden agenda – see below for examples!

4.

Do they have a hidden agenda?

Most authors or writers will have an agenda. Some agendas will be obvious, some less so. Sometimes the writer may have the best intentions at heart, and not even realize they have an agenda, but will still have one.

More obvious agendas include:

- The sale of a product or service, for instance nutritional supplements, which often try to 'scare' people into believing they can't live without them.
- Creating a catchy headline to help drive traffic to their site (then potentially earn more through paid advertising or product sales). For instance, the 'fruit is evil' headline is often used by people selling ketogenic diet plans or products.
- The desire to build a name for themselves or attract attention by posting controversial content – this is especially prevalent in the social media world.

Less obvious agendas include:

- Entrenched beliefs. For example, people who have grown up eating meat sometimes feel that veganism threatens their traditions and beliefs, and may cherry-pick studies that support their arguments. Equally, people who are passionate about veganism may wish to convince as many other people as possible to go vegan and therefore – albeit with the best intentions – may not present a balanced argument when it comes to nutrition-related topics.

- Working in an industry which they are trying to either promote or defend. An obvious example would be nutrition articles on the European Dairy Association website, which has a clear financial interest in touting the health benefits of cow's milk.

- A nutritionist who has based their entire career endorsing a particular way of eating may feel threatened by new research that contradicts them, and may keep endorsing their methods despite mounting evidence that proves them either ineffective or even dangerous. For instance, low-carbohydrate diets have been shown to be less effective for weight loss than plant-based diets.[1] Not only that, but they're in fact associated with increased mortality risk.[2] Still, many nutritionists may not wish to acknowledge the growing evidence because it contradicts the practices that they're known for.

I must admit, all this sounds rather cynical. But of course, there are many sources of information from nutritionists and writers whose main driver is genuinely to help improve the health of the reader (me included!). My hope is that bearing these four questions in mind will help you to cut through the noise and barrage of misinformation of the internet, and work out which sources you can trust.

THE DIFFERENT TYPES OF NUTRITION RESEARCH

It's also very helpful to understand what types of evidence there are. Of course, this is important to know if you're a little 'bookish' like me and enjoy doing your own search of the scientific literature. But it's also really valuable to bear this in mind when you're reading any nutrition-related article. Perhaps your friend has shared a link to a website telling you to take a new supplement for athletic performance: having a basic understanding of this is a powerful way to tell if that website is citing the best available evidence, or just cherry-picking the studies that happen to back up their argument.

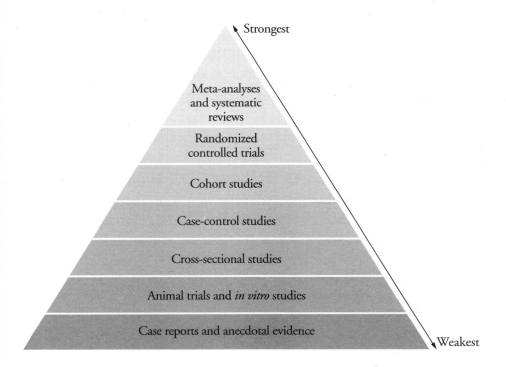

Strongest

Meta-analyses and systematic reviews

Randomized controlled trials

Cohort studies

Case-control studies

Cross-sectional studies

Animal trials and *in vitro* studies

Case reports and anecdotal evidence

Weakest

Here is what's known as the hierarchy of evidence. It lists the main forms of scientific health and nutrition research, and orders them from the weakest forms of evidence at the bottom to the strongest forms of evidence at the top. That's not to say that any one is inherently 'bad', but as you'll see, each form of evidence has strengths and weaknesses that should be taken into account when weighing up the evidence on a given topic.

- **Case reports and anecdotal evidence**

Although they're at the bottom of the pyramid, case reports can be really useful. Consider an extremely rare condition that affects one in 5 million people: it would be very difficult to gather enough people with the condition to run a controlled study, so until a larger trial can be done, anecdotal descriptions of individual cases might be the best evidence we could ask for. The same would go for a particularly specific case in sports nutrition, for example nutritional strategies for a disabled athlete (in which sports nutrition is lacking) completing a unique ultra-distance challenge. It's always worth documenting these cases in a scientific manner, because if a treatment or therapy worked well for one person, there's a chance it may work for someone else with the same rare set of circumstances.

But if we're looking at a topic that isn't rare, then why settle for anecdotal evidence of specific cases where there's a *chance* that a treatment or therapy *may* work for you, when there could be much more robust scientific research available?

Outside of the scientific literature, we're also bombarded with anecdotal cases. I've worked with many athletes who had previously based their nutrition on the advice of friends, which is commonplace among sportspeople. And just think of all the celebrities and social media influencers claiming that certain diets or products work for them, often along with 'before and after' pictures. There are likely to be many other factors at play (bear in mind the four questions above), and it doesn't necessarily mean they'll work for you too! Of course, if there's strong science behind a nutritional approach, then combining this with anecdotal evidence can be useful to help people relate to it. But anecdotal evidence alone should certainly not be taken as gospel.

• Animal trials and in vitro studies

Aside from the ethical implications of running experiments on animals, there's a significant scientific limitation when it comes to animal trials: the physiology of other animals is different to the physiology of humans. One of the best examples of this is in the research on soy foods like edamame beans, tofu and tempeh. There have, in the past, been concerns about oestrogen-like activities of the isoflavones (naturally occurring plant compounds found in soybeans) decreasing testosterone levels in men. However, the basis of these claims stem from early studies conducted on rats – and it's since been shown that rodents metabolize isoflavones quite differently to humans. In fact, a meta-analysis (more on meta-analyses later) reviewing the results from 15 controlled *human* clinical trials showed no effect of soy consumption on testosterone levels in men.[3]

In vitro studies are on the same level of this evidence hierarchy because of similar limitations. *In vitro* translates from Latin as 'in glass' because it refers to experiments carried out in laboratories, often in test tubes or petri dishes. Under laboratory conditions, isolated molecules, cells or tissues are studied closely to see how a biological mechanism might work. This is great because it allows the cells being studied to be observed much more closely, and in more detail, than if it were *in vivo* (within humans or animals).

But the downside is that *in vitro* studies don't replicate the same conditions going on inside the human body. Cells studied on a glass slide are in a very controlled and stable environment, compared to the unfathomably complex environment within the human body. They might show a mechanistic effect within cells, but that doesn't necessarily mean that'll translate into whole body physiological responses in an applied setting, such as muscle strength or endurance performance.

• Cross-sectional studies

Cross-sectional studies are observational in nature, meaning there's no experiment involved, but instead they collect information from a population at a specific point in time, usually using questionnaires or medical records. A benefit of this type of research is that it's possible to involve a large number of people relatively easily. Perhaps the most well-known example of cross-sectional analysis is a national census – data is collected from residents to give us a 'snapshot' of information about people living in the country in question.

What cross-sectional studies can do is show if there's an association between two factors: for instance, they might find a correlation between dietary quality and happiness scores. But because they only provide a 'snapshot' of information, what they can't do is prove what's causing that association.

In this example, you might assume that correlation exists because eating a higher-quality diet makes you happy. That might well be the case, but because the study was cross-sectional, it can't prove what's causing that association. It could be that how happy you are affects how you eat: if you're happier you might be more motivated to shop, prepare and eat healthier foods, and that could equally be the cause of the association. Or the cause could be bi-directional, with quality of diet and level of happiness both interacting with each other. We just can't tell from a cross-sectional study alone.

Another thing to bear in mind is that it's very difficult to account for other variables that might affect the results. In this example, there are countless socio-demographic factors, such as income, that could affect both dietary quality and happiness, so these could also be the cause of the association between the two.

• Case-control and cohort studies

Case-control and cohort studies, like cross-sectional studies, are observational – so they also collect data without interfering with or affecting the participants. However, the difference is that they both gather information *over time*. In case-control studies, researchers look back over time retrospectively, whereas cohort studies follow people going forward over time.

They therefore both have an advantage over cross-sectional studies at showing the potential cause of an association. Let's use the happiness example to illustrate this: if participants who improved their dietary quality went on, over time, to become happier, then we could say with a bit more confidence that dietary quality does affect our happiness.

The downside to these types of trials, however, is that it's still very difficult to account for all the confounding factors – other influences at play – that might affect the results. Researchers might be able to adjust for some of them (such as income, sex, and age) with their statistical models, but there are countless other possible confounding factors and biases which could affect the results, including the placebo effect, where just the belief in a treatment or therapy produces a beneficial (or detrimental) effect.

- **Randomized controlled trials**

Now we're getting to some very robust evidence, because randomized controlled trials (RCTs) do control for bias (or they at least try to). They do this by randomly assigning participants to two (or more) groups – one group is the control, and another experimental group receives a specific treatment or intervention. Ideally the control group would be given a placebo (such as a 'dud' pill) so that the participants don't know which group they're in. This helps to reduce bias – and is known as 'blinding' the trial. 'Double blinding' the trial means even the researchers don't know which participants receive the treatment, so they can't unintentionally influence the outcome (known as researcher bias).

Any differences in outcome between the groups can be more accurately attributed to whether they had the intervention: confounding factors like age, sex, income, education, health, etc. are removed because participants are randomly assigned to the different groups. The placebo effect can also be controlled for if a suitable placebo is used, because the participants don't know if they're having the treatment or not.

As with any form of experiment, there are downsides even to RCTs. Certain things can't be tested in a placebo-controlled manner – for example, it would be very difficult to conduct a double-blinded RCT for dietary quality, because the participants would probably figure out pretty quickly if they'd been assigned to the healthy or the unhealthy diet group! Cost is another factor – RCTs tend to be expensive, and to test outcomes such as diseases that might take years to manifest, would be very money- and time-consuming.

• Meta-analyses and systematic reviews

Right at the top of the pyramid, we have meta-analyses and systematic reviews, and these are considered the 'gold standard' of scientific evidence. They're not experiments in themselves, but instead they review and analyse previous experiments. Systematic reviews carefully (and systematically!) comb through the published literature on a given topic, then condense the results from numerous trials into one paper that discusses everything we know so far about that topic. Meta-analyses go one step further and use complex statistical methods to combine the data from multiple papers to give us a more specific overall picture.

Both of these help us to avoid 'single study syndrome' – the common trap of relying too heavily on any one study. Some studies published may have design flaws, outdated methodologies, or perhaps too few participants to be accurate. Therefore, it's always better to look at the general body of research rather than latching on to one or two papers, and meta-analyses and reviews do that for us, in a systematic fashion. For example, this is particularly important when considering any of the countless new supplements on the market claiming to enhance performance. I always advise carefully evaluating the evidence behind their safety and efficacy before deciding if the potential benefits outweigh any known or unknown risks. The ergogenic aids discussed in Chapter 7 all have numerous studies – mechanistic and applied meta-analyses – to show their effectiveness.

Meta-analyses often use forest plots like the one opposite to help visualize the results. This forest plot is from a meta-analysis researching the relationship between red and processed meat intake with all-cause mortality.[4] In this forest plot, squares to the right of the vertical line represent studies showing an increased risk of mortality with higher red and processed meat consumption. Squares on the left (of which there are none) would represent a protective effect. Results whose horizontal lines cross the vertical line (of which there is one) represent data that is not statistically significant. The diamond at the bottom represents the data from all these studies combined.

You can see that the diamond is very much to the right of the vertical line, showing that the body of research, when combined, clearly shows that higher red and processed meat consumption is associated with increased risk of mortality.

There was one study, however, that just crosses the vertical line, meaning it wasn't quite statistically significant. A newspaper headline or website might quote this one study, perhaps cherry-picking it to augment their case that eating more red and processed meat doesn't affect our health (single study syndrome).

So you can see how using meta-analyses and systematic reviews, where they exist, is much more reliable than quoting individual studies as they account for the whole body of scientific literature to date. Meta-analyses can combine results of observational studies (like cross-sectional, cohort or case-control studies) or, even better, randomized controlled trials, if it's a research question where they can be used.

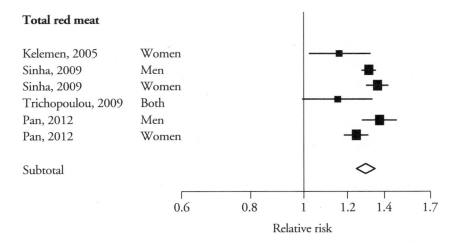

Source: Larsson and Orsini (2014)[5]

In fact, we can go one better than looking at meta-analyses alone. In an ideal world, to paint the clearest picture, we would combine evidence from more than one of these levels of evidence. For example, we have meta-analyses showing us that increased fruit and vegetable consumption is associated with decreased risk of cancer, which is very strong evidence. However, we could complement this information further with *in vitro* studies that show us several possible biological mechanisms and pathways that help to explain *how* fruit and vegetables have this protective effect. So we can use these different forms of evidence in conjunction to say with high confidence (unless stronger evidence emerges to prove otherwise) that eating more fruit and vegetables is protective against cancer. Keep an eye out for references to meta-analyses and systematic reviews throughout this book, sometimes also combined with other forms of research, to give us the clearest overall picture possible.

It should be mentioned that some researchers and statisticians spend their entire careers assessing and examining the strengths and weaknesses of the different forms of evidence. In reality, there are many subcategories within each level and some other forms of research that are less common. So, for the sake of brevity, this is a general overview of the most common forms of scientific health and nutrition research you're likely to come across. But with this general overview of some of the more common types of scientific studies, I hope you'll now feel better equipped to judge the quality of research presented to you on any given topic. For me, this is the most useful skill I've learned and developed throughout my nutrition education and training: you can learn a lot in the field of nutrition, but the science is always evolving, with new studies emerging daily, so being able to objectively assess the research and adjust your behaviours or advice accordingly is key.

CHAPTER 3

WHAT ARE THE HEALTH BENEFITS OF A VEGAN DIET?

Now we've discussed how best to weigh up the evidence, it's a good time to look at what the most robust, and latest, science shows us about the health benefits of a plant-based diet.

Doing what we can to help protect our health is important for everyone, at any stage of life. The old adage that people don't know what they've got until it's gone is perhaps most pertinent when it comes to health – it's hard to appreciate the value of being well until you're sick. Good health is also the foundation on which great sporting achievements can be built: illness can put a stop to training, temporarily or permanently, so staying healthy can mean more consistent training and even a longer sporting career. There are many more direct ways in which plant-based diets can help performance too, which we'll touch on in this chapter but will cover in much greater detail in subsequent chapters.

For now, though, we'll focus on the overall health benefits of a plant-based diet – you'll see that there's overwhelmingly strong evidence in its favour. In fact, in general, the evidence shows a stepwise reduction in risk for the most prevalent non-communicable diseases in the West as the diet becomes more plant-based: the level of protection seems to increase as we move from omnivorous, semi-vegetarian, vegetarian, through to vegan diets.

As well as seeing *how* a plant-based diet can offer such powerful health benefits, later in the chapter we'll also go on to look at *why* it has such effects. We'll unpick some of the biological mechanisms which are thought to be responsible for these effects, so we can try and adopt habits that promote these mechanisms, and in turn optimize your plant-based diet.

Acknowledging the pitfalls of nutrition research

As with the study of any whole food groups or dietary patterns, it's practically impossible to conduct randomized controlled trials (RCTs) that are placebo-controlled for vegan diets: the participants in such studies would obviously know straight away if they'd been assigned to the experimental group eating a plant-based diet, or the control group given a diet containing animal products. You can't exactly provide a 'dud' pill as a placebo for whole foods!

Therefore, much of the evidence reporting the health benefits of vegan diets comes in the form of observational research like cohort and cross-sectional studies. Enough of these observational studies have now been done across various populations in numerous countries to allow for meta-analyses of them. There have also been some meta-analyses of RCTs that aren't placebo-controlled. So, while they're not perfect, these are the best forms of evidence we could ask for. We'll also look at the mechanistic evidence to show us the possible biological pathways to explain these results – so we'll be looking at why, as well as how, a plant-based diet promotes good health by combining evidence from several different levels of the hierarchy we discussed in Chapter 2!

It can also be tricky to factor out other lifestyle factors, because vegans as a group *tend* to be more health-conscious – some studies show that vegans are less likely to smoke, or drink heavily, and are more likely to exercise, for instance.[1] This does depend on the reason behind adopting a plant-based diet: those doing so for health reasons are much more likely to implement these other healthy lifestyle choices, whereas those doing so for ethical reasons (such as animal welfare and sustainability) might not necessarily take as much care of their health.[2, 3] While studies of plant-based diets often take measures to control for these lifestyle choices in the statistical models, it can still make it difficult to assess precisely how much of the difference is down to the diet alone.

This is where evidence from Seventh-day Adventists comes in handy as additional, supporting evidence. This religious group provides a unique opportunity to compare the diets of vegans, vegetarians and meat eaters in a population with generally similar lifestyle habits. That's because the Adventist Church promotes a healthy lifestyle. Adventists are therefore generally health-conscious: they typically don't smoke or drink alcohol, and most avoid caffeine. They promote social ties through attending regular religious services. They tend to avoid junk food, and those who do eat meat typically do so at low levels.[4] Differences in health outcomes between vegans, vegetarians and meat eaters can, therefore, be more accurately attributed to those diet choices, rather than other lifestyle factors. So with the following health benefits, we'll look at meta-analyses of observational studies, RCTs (where they exist) and large studies of Adventists, combining all these forms of evidence to paint the clearest picture possible.

- Cardiovascular disease (CVD)

CVD is a class of diseases that involve the heart (cardio) or blood vessels (vascular). The most common of these are coronary artery diseases (restricted blood flow to the heart) but they also include other heart diseases, stroke (restricted blood flow to part of the brain) and peripheral artery disease (restricted blood flow elsewhere in the body).

CVDs are the leading cause of death globally. They are even more prominent in Western countries such as the UK and the US. In fact, across Europe, CVDs account for more than half of all deaths. While some cases of CVD are hereditary (passed on through our genes), the vast majority of cases (around 80%) are thought to be preventable, according to the World Health Organization.[5] This statistic never ceases to amaze me – it's astonishing to think that of the vast number of CVD cases across the world, with all the pain and devastation they cause, the majority are attributed to lifestyle factors, many of which could be modified, if only people were made aware, and had the means to do so.

The main cause of CVDs is atherosclerosis, which is the

narrowing and hardening of arteries that results in impaired blood flow and delivery of oxygen throughout the body. The diagram on page 30 shows the stages of progression of atherosclerosis, but you'll see that it always starts with damage to the endothelium, the layer of cells lining the arteries. This damage can be caused by elevated cholesterol, high blood pressure, smoking, alcohol, other toxins, and oxidative stress – many of which can be affected by modifiable lifestyle choices like diet.

It's important to remember that although the clinical manifestations of CVD, such as heart attack and stroke, usually appear from middle age, atherosclerosis has a long asymptomatic phase of development which begins early in life, often as early as childhood.[6] So it's never too early to start thinking about changing habits to protect your cardiovascular health. If you're an athlete, you may be thinking, 'Why should an active person like me worry about CVD?' Well, while there's no doubt that exercise significantly decreases the risk of CVD, athletes certainly aren't immune, and often overestimate the amount of protection that exercise affords.[7] Physical activity alone is not a fail-safe insurance policy. Periodic screening is advised for elite athletes by the International Olympic Committee,[8] because there are occasional tragedies where elite athletes and exercise enthusiasts have suffered heart attacks – you may remember some of the poignant instances of this happening during high-profile events, such as televised football matches and marathons. Yes, many of these instances are due to genetic heart abnormalities, but atherosclerotic heart disease is the leading cause of sudden cardiac death in athletes over 35 years old.[9] So other risk factors, such as cholesterol, high blood pressure and oxidative stress, all of which are strongly related to diet, can still play a pivotal role.

1. Healthy blood vessel

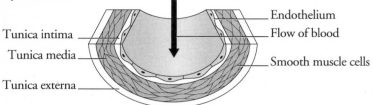

Tunica intima

Tunica media

Tunica externa

Endothelium

Flow of blood

Smooth muscle cells

2. Endothelial dysfunction

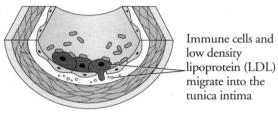

Immune cells and low density lipoprotein (LDL) migrate into the tunica intima

3. Fatty streak formation

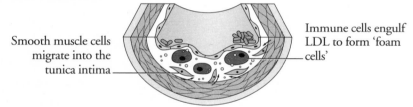

Smooth muscle cells migrate into the tunica intima

Immune cells engulf LDL to form 'foam cells'

4. Fibrous plaque atheroma

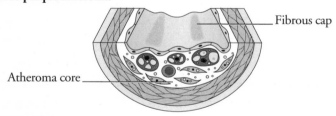

Fibrous cap

Atheroma core

5. Advanced/vulnerable plaque

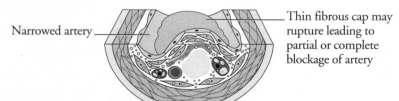

Narrowed artery

Thin fibrous cap may rupture leading to partial or complete blockage of artery

When it comes to reducing the risk of CVDs, in particular heart disease, a plant-based diet has been shown to be one of the most promising of lifestyle modifications. The largest meta-analysis to date, reviewing data from 96 observational studies, showed a striking 25% reduction in risk of ischemic heart disease in vegans and vegetarians versus omnivores.[10] Another recent meta-analysis of cohort studies showed similar results: 28% reduced incidence of coronary heart disease among plant-based diet patterns.[11] This is supported by Seventh-day Adventist studies showing reductions in risk of ischemic heart disease of 19–38% among vegetarians and vegans, which seems to be more pronounced in males than females.[12] In fact, a plant-based diet, along with other lifestyle factors such as stopping smoking, and moderate exercise, is the only diet that's been shown in smaller studies to have the potential to reverse atherosclerosis.[13]

The first of the Adventist studies – the Adventist Mortality Study – also showed a 35% reduced risk of cerebrovascular disease (such as stroke) in vegans and vegetarians.[14] But subsequent Adventist studies, as well as other prospective studies, showed no impact (positive or negative) of a plant-based diet on risk of stroke.[15,16]

The reason the evidence for protection from stroke isn't as strong as it is for heart disease could be explained by vitamin B_{12} status. Low vitamin B_{12} status is a known risk factor for stroke,[17] and as you'll see in Chapter 5, vegans are at risk of low vitamin B_{12} status if they don't supplement appropriately, because it's a nutrient that's hard to find in reliable quantities in plant foods. For example, two recent large cohort studies in Taiwan showed that a plant-based diet was accompanied by a small but meaningful reduced risk of stroke. More interestingly, though, they found that by ensuring adequate B_{12}

intake in the plant-based group, this protective effect was amplified even further.[18] This is one of many reasons why it's so important to ensure healthy B12 levels through supplementation on a plant-based diet, which we'll discuss in much greater detail in Chapter 5.

A few years ago, a client came to me because she'd recently had a medical for insurance purposes, which revealed she had high cholesterol levels, particularly high LDL (the 'bad' type of cholesterol which is a risk factor for CVD). This was unexpected and distressing for her because she was otherwise in seemingly good health – she was very lean, fit, and in fact was training for an Ironman event. On assessment of her diet, it became clear that although she incorporated lots of healthy home-cooked foods, there was a very high intake of saturated fat too. Meats, cheeses, butter and coconut oil, as well as lots of biscuits, contributed significantly to her energy intake, and she often included these foods in an attempt to match the energy demands of her high training volume. We discussed how a plant-based diet would help, and ways in which she could make healthier choices to achieve the high energy intake she required. She had further tests just two months after changing her diet, which showed a 10% reduction in LDL cholesterol while her HDL 'good' cholesterol remained unchanged. Not only that, but she saw marked improvements in her trial times and reported faster recovery from her training – as we'll see in Chapter 7, some of the same mechanisms which provide these health benefits can also be responsible for improving performance too.

• Various cancers

After cardiovascular diseases, all cancers combined are the next most important cause of death and morbidity in Europe, accounting for around 20% of deaths.[19] Cancer is the uncontrolled growth and spread of cells that arises from a change in the DNA of one single cell. That initial change may be triggered by external agents and/or inherited genetic factors, and can affect almost any part of the body.

Tobacco and alcohol consumption are the largest contributors to cancer rates, thought to cause about 40% of cases across Europe. However, it's been estimated that if the consequences of diet, obesity and inactivity are added, the percentage of cancers caused by lifestyle factors rises to about 60%.[20]

So, while genetics undoubtedly play a major role in cancer development, diet and other lifestyle factors can make a significant difference too. This is certainly supported by the research into plant-based diets. The same large meta-analysis investigating plant-based dietary patterns, reviewing 96 individual studies, showed that the incidence rate of cancer was reduced by 8% among vegetarians, and by 15% in vegans.[21] This is again consistent with findings from Adventist cohort studies which for vegetarians showed an 8% decrease in risk for all cancers combined, including a 24% lower risk of gastrointestinal cancers (such as oesophageal, stomach and colon). Again, this effect was even more prominent for vegans, with a decrease in risk of 16% for all cancers, including a 34% lower risk for female-specific cancers.[22]

A professional rugby player came to see me because of concerns he had about his family history of prostate cancer. He'd heard that a plant-based diet could help, but was concerned it might affect his performance. I wanted to make it clear that diet and lifestyle are certainly no guarantees for prevention, with age and genetics being by far the most important risk factors. That being said, making changes to reduce other modifiable risk factors would certainly help to stack the cards in his favour. At the time, he had a higher body fat percentage than he desired, and his diet contained some vegetables, the occasional piece of fruit, lots of grains, and lots of meat, dairy and eggs. He was also taking a daily multivitamin religiously. We devised a plant-based nutritional strategy to incorporate many more whole plant foods into his diet to increase intake of fibre, antioxidants, and other phytochemicals, while providing plenty of energy and protein to fuel his training and recovery. On follow-up, he had lost a little bit of weight, which he reported was helping his speed and endurance on the pitch, and blood tests showed significantly lower levels of inflammatory markers, which are known risk factors for cancer. He was feeling much less dependent on his multivitamin and, as a nice side-effect, his cholesterol levels were markedly improved too!

- Type 2 diabetes

Under normal conditions, when we eat, the energy from our food causes blood sugar levels to rise, and beta cells in the pancreas respond by producing the hormone insulin. Insulin signals to cells in our liver, fat and skeletal muscles to absorb glucose from our bloodstream, bringing blood sugar levels back down to a normal, safe, level. Diabetes is a class of metabolic disorders, where these blood sugar control mechanisms are altered, and is characterized by high blood sugar levels over a prolonged period of time, which can be harmful. Across Europe, around one in ten adults (and rising) aged over 25 years have diabetes.[23] There are two main categories:

- Type 1 diabetes is a largely genetic autoimmune disorder that damages those beta cells in the pancreas, meaning insulin production is impaired, preventing the body from adequately regulating blood sugar levels.
- Type 2 diabetes makes up the majority (90%) of diabetes cases and is thought to result initially from the body's inability to respond to insulin (known as insulin resistance). The pancreatic beta cells compensate by going into overdrive to produce more insulin, and over a prolonged period of time, sometimes years, those overworked beta cells begin to fail.

In type 2 diabetes, why does the body stop responding to insulin in the first place? Well, genetics play a role, but the main risk factors are lifestyle-related: sedentary lifestyles, smoking, being overweight, having high blood pressure, and raised cholesterol levels. So it's no surprise that changing the diet can reduce the risk of developing type 2 diabetes. In fact, plant-based diets are associated with a significant reduction in risk: a meta-analysis of cross-sectional and cohort studies showed a 27% risk reduction in developing diabetes.[24] The latest Adventist Health Study supports this reduction in risk, and also shows a stepwise effect as the population moves towards a more plant-based diet: semi-vegetarians had a 24% lower risk, pescatarians 30%, vegetarians 46%, and vegans 49% reduced risk, even after adjusting for factors such as age, sex, income, BMI, and television watching.[25] Another large study of Adventists had even more pronounced results: 38% reduced risk in vegetarians and 62% reduced risk in vegans.[26]

Again, athletes as a group are at lower risk of developing type 2 diabetes, but are not immune to it. Regular exercise lowers many risk factors for diabetes, such as fasting insulin and glucose levels, blood pressure and body weight,[27] but there are many examples of elite level athletes developing type 2 diabetes, which can then impede athletic performance, for example by reducing peak exercise capacity (VO2 max).[28] Combining the beneficial effects of exercise with a plant-based diet can provide an even greater reduction in risk for type 2 diabetes.

• Dementia

Dementia is an umbrella term that covers a wide range of diseases and conditions, characterized by a decline in memory, language and problem-solving. These functions are vital in order to perform everyday activities and live an independent life, and a progression of dementia can also have a devastating effect on behaviours, feelings and relationships.

Alzheimer's disease is the most common cause of dementia. Since 2001, Public Health England have reported that deaths from dementia and Alzheimer's have dramatically increased by 60% in males and have doubled in females. Part of this increase can be explained by the fact that the population of the UK is ageing and that there's an increase in awareness of dementia. Still, its prevalence worldwide is expected to double every 20 years, and it's already the leading cause of dependency and disability among older people.[29]

Genetics play a big part in determining the risk of developing dementia. But equally significant in influencing its onset are lifestyle choices – for example smoking, alcohol and sedentary lifestyles are known risk factors, while exercise, mental stimulation, strong social connections, and of course healthy diet have been shown to be protective.

Studies show higher meat consumption significantly increases risk of dementia, as evidenced by a systematic review of evidence from numerous countries in Africa, Asia, and North and South America.[30] There's also evidence from the Adventist Health Study 1 which showed that people who ate meat were twice as likely to develop dementia as their vegetarian counterparts, and the effect was exaggerated further to triple when past meat consumption was also taken into account.[31] At the same time, there is robust evidence linking higher consumption of fruit and vegetables, as is common with plant-based diets, with a protective effect. In a meta-analysis of nine cohort and cross-sectional studies, there was a 20% reduced risk of cognitive impairment and dementia with higher intake of fruit and vegetables.[32]

One point worth mentioning is that most studies also show the protective effect of fish consumption on risk of dementia.[33, 34] A key nutrient in fish that is most likely to be responsible for this effect are omega-3 fatty acids, which we cover in detail in Chapter 5, and which as you will see are easily obtained on a well-planned vegan diet.

• Longevity

With all the above evidence in mind, it may be no surprise that many studies show that a plant-based diet is also associated with living longer. The latest Adventist Health Study, assessing over 70,000 Adventists, showed all-cause mortality risk (that means dying by any cause) was reduced by 9% in vegetarians and 15% in vegans.[35] Similar results were found in a cohort of over 12,000 middle-aged adults in the US after adjusting for other important factors, showing that a plant-based diet was associated with 11% lower risk of all-cause mortality.[36]

Studies looking at the intake of components of the diet support this too: a meta-analysis of nine cohort studies showed that a higher consumption of red and processed meat was associated with a 29% increase risk of all-cause mortality.[37] On the other hand, a large meta-analysis reviewing 95 studies showed that for every 200g of fruit and vegetables added to the diet daily, there was a 10% reduction in all-cause mortality, even up to 800g (approx. 10 portions of fruit and veg).[38]

To report an honest representation of the literature, it's important to point out, however, that not all studies have shown a difference in longevity. For example, the same large meta-analysis quoted earlier in the chapter, which showed a reduction in risk of cancer and heart disease among plant-based diets, didn't actually find a difference in all-cause mortality.[39] Another cohort in the UK of over 60,000 adults showed no significant difference in all-cause mortality between vegans, vegetarians and meat eaters.[40]

All the evidence we've covered so far certainly shows that a plant-based diet decreases risk of the most prevalent diseases in the developed world. This suggests that even if there were no difference in overall lifespan between vegans and omnivores, it could at least delay the onset of disease, a concept that Dr James Fries, Professor of Medicine at Stanford University, coined as the 'compression of morbidity'. The first diagram below shows the lifespan of someone living to the age of around 90 years. Thanks to the wonders of modern medicine, they've been able to live a long life. But as you can see, many of those years were spent living with chronic illness, taking medication, and perhaps with resulting impacts on life choices, emotions and relationships. The second diagram shows someone living to the same age, but with significant postponement of the same chronic diseases. So even if vegans didn't live longer, the onset of disease is likely to at least be delayed. They are able to enjoy many more active, healthy years because the period of morbidity has been compressed towards the end of their life.

For athletes and sportspeople, this could mean a longer

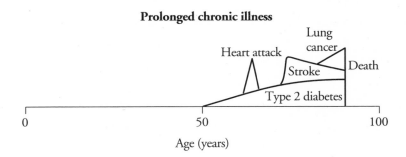

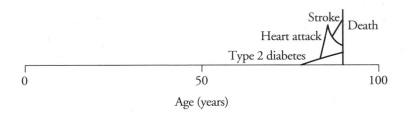

career, and enjoying many active years even after retirement from professional competition. In this sense, I like to think of healthy plant-based diets as having the ability to add life to your years, as well as potentially adding years to your life.

The blame game

As we've seen, lifestyle factors such as diet have a significant impact on disease risk. But even someone living the healthiest of lives can get ill. I want to take this opportunity to point out that no one should ever feel that it's their 'fault' for getting ill – genetics still play a huge role and there are many environmental factors outside our control. Just remember, an illness does not define you as a person, and what makes up someone's character is about so much more than just their health. I do think it's really important that more people are made aware of the impact of lifestyle and diet choices, but recognize that we need to tackle the individual 'blame' culture that exists surrounding ill-health. Not only does this place unnecessary stress and stigma on those dealing with disease, it also absolves government, health bodies and big business from taking responsibility for our health.

WHY DOES A PLANT-BASED DIET REAP ALL THESE BENEFITS?

The meta-analyses discussed above clearly show the beneficial effects a plant-based diet can have on the risk factors for the most prevalent non-communicable diseases. It's important to also look at *why* they have these effects, by looking at the possible biological pathways – taking a closer look at the mechanisms within the body by which plant-based diets reap all these health rewards. Remember, to understand *why* as well as *how* a plant-based diet can offer such protection helps us to paint the clearest possible picture of the evidence.

Well, the mechanisms behind why a plant-based diet results in these incredible health benefits can be broadly divided into two main categories:

1.

Vegans tend to eat more whole plant foods

Studies show that vegans tend to eat more whole plant foods.[41] But we don't need studies to tell us that – it also makes common sense: if you don't eat meat or animal products, you need to replace those calories with other foods, and often these are whole plant foods. For example, an omnivore might have roast chicken with their Sunday roast, whereas a vegan would typically replace it with a nut roast made with pulses, vegetables and nuts, adding further to their intake of whole plant foods. A beefburger would likely be replaced with a patty made from beans and vegetables. Vegan curries often contain various vegetables and pulses such as chickpeas, versus a typical omnivorous order consisting just of chicken in a curry sauce. Even pizzas tend to be topped with colourful vegetables rather than just cheese and pepperoni.

Of course, not all vegans eat more plants – with today's meat-free alternatives, it's now possible to live off cheap ready meals and junk food as a vegan. But remember that the studies quoted in this section are based on *averages at a population level*. And studies show that, *on average*, vegans do eat significantly more of these whole plant foods and have healthier dietary quality scores.

Why is this important? Well, let's look at the biological pathways by which eating more whole plant foods like fruits, vegetables, whole grains, pulses, nuts and seeds can drastically and significantly improve health.

Antioxidants

To appreciate the importance of antioxidants, we must first understand how free radicals work. Atoms are made up of a central nucleus made of protons and neutrons, which have electrons surrounding them in orbit. These electrons usually exist in pairs, but various environmental and metabolic factors can cause an atom or molecule to 'lose' an electron, causing it to become a free radical which is highly unstable: when it encounters another molecule it looks to 'scavenge' an electron to match up with its unpaired electron, causing that neighbouring molecule to become a free radical itself. The newly produced free radical then looks to scavenge another electron, and so on. This process continues in a chain reaction which can result in the damaging of protein molecules, unsaturated fatty acids, and even DNA.

Free radicals are constantly produced by the body, especially through processes that involve an oxidation reaction – such as those required for energy production. They can also be useful – for example, they're involved in several cell signalling pathways, and some immune cells use free radicals to fight infection. However, your body needs to keep the free radical balance in check, as long-term elevated levels can cause serious harm to the body.

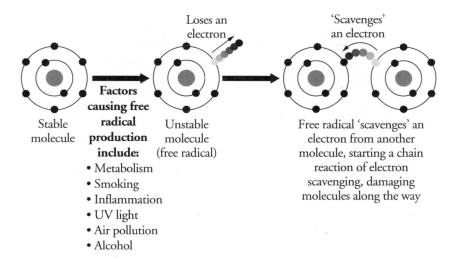

Stable molecule → **Factors causing free radical production include:**
- Metabolism
- Smoking
- Inflammation
- UV light
- Air pollution
- Alcohol

Loses an electron → Unstable molecule (free radical)

'Scavenges' an electron → Free radical 'scavenges' an electron from another molecule, starting a chain reaction of electron scavenging, damaging molecules along the way

In fact, chronic oxidative stress from elevated free radical levels can be shown to be one of the primary causes for all the major diseases listed earlier in this chapter: it's linked with the development of CVD,[42] cancer,[43] type 2 diabetes,[44] and dementia.[45] From a fitness perspective, increased free radical production can also lead to skeletal muscle atrophy (muscle wasting) during periods of inactivity which can reduce strength and power, and therefore negatively impact performance.[46]

This is where antioxidants come in, as they have a wonderful ability to stabilize and quench free radicals. They work either by generously donating an electron to free radicals, often becoming oxidized and inactive in the process and without becoming a free radical themselves (thereby interrupting that chain reaction of oxidative stress) or by breaking down the free radical molecule to render it harmless.

The body can generate its own antioxidants as part of its free radical defence system, but some must also come from the diet – for example beta-carotene and vitamins C and E.

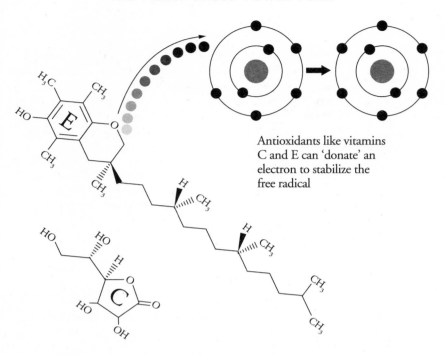

Antioxidants like vitamins C and E can 'donate' an electron to stabilize the free radical

There are also nutrients in food that are needed as part of the body's own free radical defence system (such as copper and selenium), and there are numerous other non-essential antioxidants occurring in food that we can survive without, but including them provides significant benefits to general health.

There are some antioxidants in meat and animal products, but a comprehensive review of the antioxidant properties of over 3,000 foods worldwide showed that plant foods have an average of **64 times** the antioxidant properties of animal-based foods.[47] Therefore, the higher antioxidant intake when eating more whole plant foods can help prevent oxidative stress, and is one of the pathways by which eating more plants can provide such a profound protective effect against so many major diseases.

What about antioxidant supplements?

As we'll see in Chapters 6 and 7, the rich antioxidant content of whole plant foods is a key mechanism that helps to improve not only health, but exercise performance and recovery too. Many clients I see, from recreationally active people to elite athletes, ask me about taking antioxidant supplements as a simple way to recreate these effects. But, when taken in supplement form, antioxidant supplements have been shown to blunt the body's adaptation to exercise[48] and there's no evidence they improve health outcomes.[49] In fact, recent meta-analyses show that supplementing with the antioxidants beta-carotene and vitamin E can *increase* our risk of death,[50] and the same goes for higher doses of vitamin A.[51] Not exactly the health benefits you might expect!

This might sound quite bizarre, because we know we need antioxidants in our diet. Well, the reason is that when we get these nutrients naturally through whole foods, we're eating so much more than specific, singular nutrients in isolation, like we do when we take supplements. For example, fruit and vegetables contain countless protective bioactive compounds, including antioxidants but also vitamins, minerals, proteins, fibre, fats and other phytonutrients. There are thousands of these compounds that we've identified, and many more we don't even know about yet. These compounds interact with each other through numerous, complex mechanisms within the body, resulting in some incredible health benefits. Taking antioxidants in supplement form simply can't replicate the complexity of whole plant foods.

Gut health

The gut microbiome is one of the most fascinating and rapidly developing areas of human health research. It's estimated that the human body is made of approximately 30–40 trillion cells.[52] Recent research has uncovered the mindblowing fact that the number of microorganisms in and on our bodies (mostly bacteria but also including fungi, viruses and other microbes) outnumbers our own body's cells by around 10 to 1. Because these microbes are much smaller than human cells, they only make up around 1–3% of our total body weight.[53] So for example, a person weighing 70kg could be carrying 1–2kg of bacteria!

We have microorganisms all over us – our mouths, noses, hair, skin and genitalia – but most are contained within our gut, which is known as the gut microbiome. Here, they play a crucial role in allowing us to digest food and absorb nutrients that otherwise would be unavailable to us. Some of these microbes also produce beneficial compounds, such as vitamins, and anti-inflammatory compounds that our bodies can't make ourselves. So it's a prime example of a mutually beneficial symbiotic relationship – we look after our bacteria by feeding them and providing a warm, cosy environment in our gut, and in return they help us break down many of the proteins, lipids and carbohydrates in our diet into nutrients we can absorb, as well as producing other compounds crucial for our survival. The gut microbiome is so important it's often referred to as the 'forgotten organ'.

What role does a plant-based diet have in improving our gut health? Well, studies show that vegans tend to have a gut microbiota which is quite distinct from that of omnivores. They're likely to have a reduced abundance of pathogenic ('bad') bacteria and a greater abundance of protective species.[54] This is mostly down to the increased fibre intake of a typical vegan diet.

Why is the higher fibre intake typical of a plant-based diet so critical? Fibres are the primary energy source for most of our healthy gut microbes, so intake can directly benefit those 'good' bacterial species.[55] Many good bacteria species also ferment certain fibres, and in the process produce short chain fatty acids (SCFAs), some of which are the main source of energy for colonocytes (the cells lining the colon) and can help keep these cells healthy, reducing risk of colon cancer through several mechanisms.[56]

SCFAs also lower the pH of the gut, which in itself inhibits the growth of pathogenic bacteria and increases the absorption of some nutrients. They've also been shown to improve the junctions between the cells lining our gut, known as the intestinal barrier, thereby reducing the absorption of pathogens and toxins, while preserving the ability to absorb nutrients.[57] So it's no surprise that SCFAs can improve other bowel disorders such as ulcerative colitis and Crohn's disease, and may reduce risk of other inflammatory diseases, type 2 diabetes, obesity and heart disease.[58] So encouraging the maintenance of a healthy gut microbiome is another key mechanism by which a plant-based diet can have such profound health benefits.

Healthy weight promotion

Around two-thirds of adults in the UK are either overweight (36%) or obese (29%).[59] This is of huge interest from a health perspective because being overweight is a significant risk factor for all the chronic diseases discussed earlier in this chapter (heart disease, cancer, type 2 diabetes and dementia), as well as many other health issues including liver disease, stroke and impaired bone health.

For many sports, especially where athletes must move their own body mass or compete within weight divisions, it's also often beneficial to achieve relatively low body fat levels. This can help improve an athlete's power to weight ratio, which can increase speed, agility, and achieve a lower energy cost of movement.

Weight gain is far too often radically oversimplified, when in fact it's a hugely complex issue. For example, genetics have increasingly been shown to play an integral role in people's appetite, and therefore weight. Also, the world around us massively influences our ability to maintain a healthy weight: accessibility of affordable healthy foods (or lack of), food culture, increasingly automated physical environments, and the constant bombardment of advertising and cheap pricing of fast food and sugary snacks and drinks. Stress, social factors, and poor sleep have all also been shown to influence food choices.

We'll discuss why traditional weight loss diets simply don't work in the long run in further detail in Chapter 9. Put simply, though, they focus so much on the sole goal of weight reduction, that they neglect to consider all these other complex factors that influence not only weight, but other important aspects of health and wellbeing too.

In comparison, a plant-based diet has been shown to both help prevent weight gain in the first place, as well as improve weight reduction in overweight populations. For example, a study of 60,000 people in the Adventist Health Study assessed body mass index (BMI), a rough measure of body weight that accounts for height, albeit still not a perfect measure, as it doesn't account for things like muscle mass. Nonetheless, they found that on average, vegans had the lowest BMI, followed incrementally by vegetarians, pescatarians, semi-vegetarians, then omnivores.[60] Similar results from a meta-analysis of observational studies reported significantly lower BMIs in those eating a plant-based diet.[61]

Plant-based diets can be far more effective for weight loss, too. A meta-analysis comparing plant-based diets with other diet approaches such as the Atkins diet and even the American Diabetes Association recommended diet showed significantly greater weight reduction in vegetarian, and even more so in vegan diets.[62] There's a whole host of reasons why plant-based diets can be so effective both for maintaining a healthy weight and for weight reduction in those looking to lose body fat. These range from psychological factors such as motives and adherence (vegan diets tends to be a long-term lifestyle choice rather than a short-lived weight-loss diet), to biological factors such as the fibre content and nutrient/calorie density of plant foods.

We'll discuss these mechanisms in more detail in Chapter 9, along with proven strategies for effective, healthy weight management. For now, though, it's useful to consider that plant-based diets can help with weight control, which can be a big advantage in many sports and activities, and can in turn reduce risk factors for cardiovascular disease, cancers, diabetes, dementia, and many other long-term health conditions.

2.

Vegans don't eat meat, eggs and dairy

This second category of reasons explaining why vegans tend to experience the profound health benefits described above might seem an obvious one. But it's an important one too. While I prefer not to dwell on the negative health effects of eating meat and animal products, I do feel it's important to consider the science of this aspect too. That's because, while there's no question that eating more fruit and vegetables is a good strategy for everyone, regardless of whether or not they

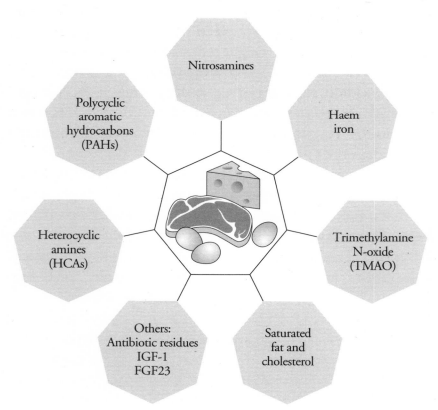

eat meat, there's also evidence to suggest that the process of eliminating meat and animal products is also an important factor in the equation when assessing the health benefits of a vegan diet. Let's discuss just some of the identified pathways that show how and why eating meat and animal products can contribute to the onset and development of several chronic diseases.

Haem iron

The iron found in plant foods comes in the form of non-haem iron, whereas meat and animal products contain haem iron. While both forms provide the body with the iron it needs, they have different structures and are absorbed differently in the gut. Higher intake of haem iron from meat is associated with increased risk of several cancers of the gastrointestinal tract, including cancers of the oesophagus, stomach,[63] and colon.[64] A primary mechanism by which haem iron increases the risk of these cancers is thought to be because it acts as a catalyst within the gastrointestinal tract for the production of N-nitroso compounds, which are potent carcinogens.[65] Haem iron can also promote the production of free radicals, which as we discussed above can cause oxidative stress, damaging various cell structures including DNA.[66]

Nitrosamines

Processed meats, such as ham, bacon, sausages, salami, hot dogs, corned beef and canned meat often contain added nitrites and nitrates, which are used to preserve the meat, particularly to prevent the overgrowth of bacteria that produce toxins caus-ing botulism — a life-threatening condition which can cause paralysis. They're also added to enhance flavour, and impart the 'desirable' pink colour of these meats. Nitrates and nitrites also occur naturally in fruit and vegetables, which, as we'll cover in Chapter 7, can be extremely healthy and aid performance. However, in processed meats, the nitrites react with the amines in the meat during processing, curing, storage and cooking to form nitrosamines, which are known potent carcinogens.[67] A meta-analysis of 49 studies showed that high intake of nitrosamines was associated with a 34% increased risk of stomach cancer[68] and could be one of the key reasons why processed meat consumption is linked with colorectal cancer.[69] The evidence is so strong that the World Health Organization have classified processed meat as a group 1 carcinogen, which is the same category as tobacco smoking and asbestos. That doesn't mean it's as dangerous as these other carcinogens, but does mean that the strength of scientific evidence is also in the highest category[70] (incidentally, unprocessed red meat is classified as a group 2A carcinogen, meaning the evidence is still strong but not quite as strong as for processed meat).

TMAO

Health and nutrition researchers used to think that red meat increased risk of heart disease just because it was high in saturated fat. But recent research has discovered another possible pathway – through a substance produced during the digestion and metabolism of choline, a water-soluble compound found in abundance in red meat, poultry, fish and eggs. While we do need some choline in our diet, the moderate amounts found in various grains, pulses, vegetables and fruit provide plenty for those eating a balanced vegan diet. Eaten in excess, however, bacteria in the gut feast on choline, and in doing so they produce a substance called trimethyl-amine (TMA). This is transported to the liver, where it's con-verted to trimethylamine N-oxide (TMAO). Higher blood levels of TMAO induce inflammation throughout the body, which is why it's linked with several different chronic dis-eases.[71] Recent research shows an association between higher levels of TMAO and a 23% increased risk in CVDs,[72] an 89% increased risk of type 2 diabetes[73] and links with Alzheimer's disease.[74] In fact, higher TMAO levels are associated with a 55% increased risk in all-cause mortality.[75]

Saturated fat and cholesterol

There's been huge debate over the role of saturated fat – high in meat, cheese and eggs, as well as in coconut and palm oils – on human health. A meta-analysis of observational studies from 2010 somewhat muddied the waters by conclud-ing that saturated fat intake had no association with risk of cardiovascular disease.[76] However, the researchers them-selves acknowledged that they didn't have enough informa-tion to assess what the participants were eating to replace the saturated fat in the diet. For instance, they could have been reducing their intake of saturated fat from meat and butter, but replacing those calories with sugar-laden snacks and highly processed foods, which promote weight gain and therefore also affect heart health.

However, hundreds of trials that directly fed people dif-ferent fats show with near-certainty that saturated fats in the diet reliably raise blood cholesterol levels, especially low-density lipoprotein (LDL) – the 'bad' cholesterol.[77] This is a known risk factor for cardiovascular disease. And a more recent 2015 meta-analysis of RCTs (remember – a more robust form of research than the observational studies assessed in the 2010 review) directly demonstrated this effect. It showed that reducing dietary saturated fat, especially when replaced with unsaturated fats, lowered the risk of cardiovascular events by a significant 17%.[78]

Besides the increased risk of CVD, higher intake of saturated fat also triggers a pro-inflammatory response.[79] Excessive or inappropriate inflammation plays a pivotal role in the onset and progression of atherosclerosis and can lead to other diseases related to chronic inflammation such as rheumatoid arthritis and Crohn's disease.[80] Recent research also shows that high saturated fat intake may negatively affect our gut microbiota – which as we know is paramount to our overall health.[81]

HCAs and PAHs

When meats are cooked at high temperatures, such as pan-frying or grilling, certain compounds are formed including heterocyclic amines (HCAs) and polycyclic aromatic hydrocarbons (PAHs) which have both been found to be mutagenic – i.e. they cause changes in our cells' DNA that may increase risk of cancer.[82] HCAs form when amino acids, sugars and creatine (found in muscle) react at high temperatures. PAHs form when the fat and juices from meat cause flames and smoke on grills or barbecues, which stick to the surface of the meat, and are also found in smoked meats as well as car exhaust fumes and cigarette smoke. A meta-analysis of 39 studies found a dose-response relationship between these meat-cooking related mutagens and cancer, i.e. the higher the intake of HCAs, the greater the risk of cancer (specifically colorectal cancer).[83]

This isn't an exhaustive list of the possible detrimental effects of eating meat and animal products. There are likely to be other factors at play, such as potential antibiotic residues in meat, dairy and egg products[84] which can disrupt our gut microbiome, and the proteins in animal products promoting the excessive production of certain hormones like IGF-1, which is thought to be linked with several cancers.[85, 86] This section is not designed to shock you into ditching meat and animal products. But it's important to discuss these possible mechanisms which help explain the rewards of a plant-based diet. Of course, everyone, vegan or not, can benefit from eating more whole plant foods, but it seems that reducing or eliminating meat and animal products is an equally important part of the equation.

Being vegan doesn't automatically mean being healthy!

It's important to highlight that adopting a vegan diet doesn't automatically mean you'll be blessed with good health and longevity! There are hundreds of other factors that influence health that are both somewhat within our control (such as levels of exercise, quantity and quality of sleep, and stress management techniques) and largely out of our control (including genetics, pollution exposure, healthcare availability), which have all been shown to play important roles in the development of chronic diseases.

What's more, not all vegan diets are equal. As with any type of diet, there are healthier and less healthy ways of eating that might be influenced by motivation, time constraints, or social and economic factors. I personally know some vegans who, for various reasons, rely heavily on vegan junk food, takeaways and ready meals. But I know many others who have a balanced, varied, well-planned vegan diet, based mostly around whole plant foods, all of which can be simple, inexpensive, and easy to prepare.

The purpose of this book is to help you feel informed, inspired, and equipped with the information you need to flourish on your plant-based diet and help you on your journey to good health, fitness, and longevity. A key mission of mine is to help ensure you fall into the category of vegans eating a varied, balanced, well-planned diet that you need to thrive and so you, too, can reap the substantial health rewards of the diet. Not only that, I want you to feel energetic, strong and resilient, and to out-perform the competition by taking advantage of the numerous performance and recovery benefits a plant-based diet can bring too.

CHAPTER 4

ARE VEGANS MORE PRONE TO NUTRITIONAL DEFICIENCIES?

We've looked at some of the most significant health advantages of a plant-based diet, which include reduced risk of some of the most prevalent and important diseases in the West. And, as we've seen, the evidence to support these health benefits is the best we could ask for – combining meta-analyses, randomized controlled trials, large cohort studies uniquely suited to studying vegan diets, plus what we know from mechanistic research showing us the biological pathways behind it all. Then there's the numerous ways in which a plant-based diet can help with performance for sportspeople and athletes too, as we'll discuss throughout the following chapters.

Plant-based diets were once met with scepticism, but now governments and national health bodies are beginning to acknowledge this growing body of evidence: the World Health Organization now recommends putting an emphasis on plant-based foods while limiting red and processed meat to promote human health and protect the environment; the British Dietetic Association confirms that a well-planned vegan diet can support healthy living in people of all ages (including in pregnancy, infancy and old age); as does the British Nutrition Foundation, which states that vegan diets can be nutritious and healthy.

Still, so many people I speak with have bought into the belief that we need meat and animal products in our diet to be healthy, fit and strong. I can even recall several conversations with health professionals, expressing their concern that vegans are likely to become ill due to deficiencies. While it's true that for vegans there are some key nutrients that are undoubtedly important to consider, you'll see in the next chapter just how easy it is to incorporate them into the diet. Still, this disproportionate emphasis on potential deficiencies for vegans is enough to make people cautious about giving a plant-based diet a go, despite all the mounting evidence of the health, performance and recovery benefits.

In reality, the truth is all populations have key nutrients they ought to be mindful of. For example:

- Over 50s are at higher risk of deficiencies in several nutrients, for example vitamin B_{12}, due to decreased absorption associated with ageing: in America it's recommended that all over-50s take a vitamin B_{12} supplement.

- The UK government recommends *everyone* consider taking a vitamin D supplement, especially during the winter months.

- Prior to conception and during early pregnancy, all women in the UK are advised to supplement with folic acid.

- Athletes and fitness enthusiasts may benefit from supplementation, for example consuming protein shakes or bars is common among strength training athletes, or taking carbohydrate gels in endurance events to enhance performance and recovery.

- Those taking medications may experience drug–food interactions that affect the absorption or metabolism of certain nutrients, requiring supplementation to rectify imbalances.

- Women with high menstrual losses, where it's advised the most practical way to meet iron needs is with a supplement.[1]

Most people fall into at least one of these categories. In fact, around half the UK population say they regularly take food supplements or vitamins, with a further third of people saying they've taken them in the past.[2] That's more than 8 out of 10 people in the UK who have taken, or regularly take, vitamin or food supplements. And supplement use is even higher among athletes – up to 82% of elite athletes report the regular use of sports supplements, most commonly protein drinks or bars.[3]

In fact, although it wasn't categorized in the above research into supplement use, everyone who eats bread in the UK *technically* takes a form of supplement. That's because almost all wheat flour and bread produced in the UK must, by law (Bread and Flour Regulations, 1998), be fortified with four vitamins and minerals: thiamine (vitamin B_1), niacin (vitamin B_3), calcium, and iron. This is with the exception of wholemeal flour and wheat malt flour. This law was introduced in

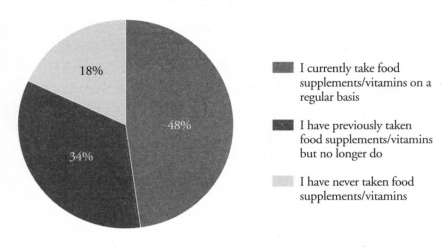

an attempt to address the widespread deficiencies in these nutrients observed across the country.

So, with the majority of people in the UK taking supplements, why is there such a big emphasis on vegans requiring supplementation? Why isn't the focus on the powerful overall health benefits of the diet, such as those covered in Chapter 3, rather than just a few isolated nutrients?

Another important question is this: why is there so rarely any focus on nutrients that vegans are *less* likely to be deficient in? As this is so often overlooked, I want to highlight a few of these nutrients here to discuss their importance.

- Fibre

We discussed in Chapter 3 why fibre is so important for maintaining a healthy weight and nurturing a healthy gut microbiome, and how both these factors, in turn, positively influence the health and functioning of almost every other system within the human body. Maintaining a lower body fat percentage can also contribute to success in various sports too.

The recommended intake of fibre for adults in the UK, both male and female, is 30g per day.* On average, Brits consume an average of just 18g a day.[4] That's only a little over half the recommended amount. Meanwhile, studies show that vegans consume an average of 41–47g of fibre a day.[5,6] This may come as no surprise, especially when you consider that fibre comes exclusively from plants, with zero fibre found in meat and animal products like milk, cheese and eggs. When you look at the table on page 62, it's easy to see how consuming a plant-based diet can help you meet your fibre intake: whole plant foods like legumes, vegetables, whole grains, fruit, nuts and seeds are brimming with both soluble and insoluble fibres.

Many people still underestimate the importance of fibre for health. I've heard far too many people say to me, 'I go to the loo regularly enough; I don't need more fibre in my diet!' But, as we've already discussed in Chapter 3, getting enough fibre is about so much more than just keeping your bowel movements regular (although that's very important too). It's also about feeding the microbes in your gut, which in turn produce many important compounds, including those all-important short-chain fatty acids. Remember, these SCFAs are the main source of energy for the cells lining your colon, so are vital for keeping your gut healthy, but they also enter

* The reference nutrient intakes discussed in this book are for adult males and females. For a comprehensive list of recommended intakes, including for pregnancy, breast feeding, children and older adults, see the British Nutrition Foundation tables using the following link: https://www.nutrition.org.uk/healthyliving/resources/nutritionrequirements.html.

FOOD	SERVING SIZE	TYPICAL FIBRE (g)
Brown lentils, cooked	1 cup	16.3
Black beans, cooked	1 cup	15.0
Broccoli, boiled	1 cup	5.2
Whole wheat pasta, cooked	1 cup	4.9
Apple, fresh	1 medium	4.4
Oats, cooked	1 cup	4.0
Raspberries, fresh	½ cup	4.0
Carrot, chopped	1 cup	3.6
Almonds, raw	28g	3.4
Sunflower seeds	28g	2.4

(Data from USDA FoodData Central https://fdc.nal.usda.gov.)

your bloodstream and play a crucial role in just about every other system in the body.

Several meta-analyses have also studied the effect of fibre on risk of cardiovascular disease, and an umbrella review of these meta-analyses (effectively a meta-analysis of meta-analyses) showed a significant reduction in risk of cardiovascular disease when comparing highest vs lowest intake of fibre.[7] The same review assessed dietary fibre's effects on cholesterol, which showed that it significantly reduces total and low-density lipoprotein (the 'bad' type) cholesterol – which is a likely key mechanism of that reduced risk of CVD.

There's another bonus to eating plenty of fibre-rich plant foods too. We've discussed how dietary antioxidants play such an important role in human health by counteracting oxidative stress and preventing numerous chronic diseases. But the fruits highest in antioxidants are not necessarily those that lead to the highest concentrations of antioxidants in the blood or target tissues.[8] That's at least partly down to the fibre content of these foods. Fibre helps to slow the absorption of antioxidants from our food, resulting in the continuous presence of a relatively low concentration of anti-oxidant compounds, which may have a greater potential benefit for the body's defence than the spike of blood anti-oxidant concentration observed immediately after ingestion of a food rich in free antioxidant compounds,[9] such as those found in antioxidant supplements or fruit juices. As we'll discuss in Chapters 6 and 7, the high antioxidant intake of healthy plant-based diets could be a key advantage to athletic performance and recovery, so this is of particular interest in a sports setting.

So, with dietary fibre keeping our bowel movements regu-lar, helping us maintain a healthy weight, aiding with the slower absorption of antioxidants, reducing cardiovascular disease risk by actively lowering our cholesterol, and provid-ing fuel for our gut microbes to produce vital compounds for our colon and elsewhere in the body, you can see why fibre is really the unsung hero of the nutrition world and certainly shouldn't be underestimated, providing a key advantage to those on a plant-based diet.

- Folate

Folate (vitamin B9) plays an essential role in numerous mech-anisms in the human body. Perhaps one of the most vital of these is its involvement in the formation of DNA and RNA (the genetic make-up of our cells), meaning it's crucial for

63

healthy cell division and production. Because red blood cells are replaced and produced at such a rapid rate, these are often the first to be affected by a folate deficiency, which if left unchecked can lead to a form of anaemia, a blood disorder in which the number of healthy red blood cells is lower than normal. Because red blood cells transport oxygen around the body, anaemia limits the amount of oxygen delivered to your tissues and organs – this means the muscles aren't getting the oxygen they require to function at their best. For endurance athletes, the red blood cells have a significantly higher turnover rate due to the stresses of training, so getting enough folate is of particular importance.[10]

The recommended intake for adult men and women in the UK is 200μg a day. The exception to this is women in the early stages of pregnancy, when it's important to take the recommended level of 400μg a day of folic acid (the man-made form of folate) as a supplement. In fact, the NHS advise that all women who are trying for a baby, and even women who *could* get pregnant, should supplement with folic acid, so that it's taken for at least one month prior to conception, through to 12 weeks of pregnancy, to ensure adequate levels during the baby's early development, and reduce risk of developing neural tube defects.[11]

Folate deficiency among adults is relatively uncommon, with around 7% of adults with evidence of low blood folate levels and indicative of risk of anaemia (but as high as 28% in 11–18 year olds).[12] Still, results from a large cohort study showed that vegans in the UK consume an average of 23% more folate than omnivores.[13] That's because a healthy plant-based diet is rich in legumes and dark green leafy vegetables, which are some of the best sources of folate (as well as most of the B vitamins). In fact, scientists first discovered folate in green leafy vegetables, and that's how it got its name: the word folate is derived from the Latin word for leaf, *folium*.

FOOD	SERVING SIZE	TYPICAL FOLATE (µg)
Edamame beans, cooked	1 cup	482
Brown lentils, cooked	1 cup	358
Pinto beans, cooked	1 cup	294
Spinach, cooked	1 cup	263
Black beans, cooked	1 cup	256
Asparagus, cooked	1 cup	243
Kidney beans, cooked	1 cup	230
Spring greens, cooked	1 cup	177
Broccoli, cooked	1 cup	168
Chickpeas, cooked	1 cup	161

(Data from USDA FoodData Central https://fdc.nal.usda.gov.)

You can see from the table just how easy it is to get 200mcg of folate a day on a plant-based diet rich in greens and pulses, as many of these foods will contribute the full amount of daily folate in just one portion. There's also folate in varying amounts in most other fruits and vegetables, including beetroot, bananas and citrus fruits, as well as nuts and seeds. Vegan women should nonetheless still follow the government advice that **all women** should supplement with folic acid prior to conception and through to 12 weeks of pregnancy.

• Potassium

Potassium is the third most abundant mineral in the body, and its importance for human health is all too often underestimated. It's classified as an electrolyte because it produces positively charged ions when dissolved in water. Molecular pumps within cell walls pull potassium into cells, and push negatively charged sodium ions out into the surrounding fluid, creating a chemical battery that drives the transmission of signals along nerves and powers the contractions of muscles. Potassium and sodium also help the kidneys to work properly, are important for energy production and fluid balance, and recent research is beginning to uncover their roles in bone health too. All these factors are key for overall health but also play important roles in performance too.

The problem with most Western diets is that they're very often far too high in sodium (found in salt) and too low in potassium (found in abundance in plant foods like greens and legumes). Some research suggests that our ancestors consumed over 11,000mg of potassium a day, mostly from plant foods, while getting under 700mg of sodium.[14] Similar intakes are found among remote tribal populations unaffected by Western influences. That's a ratio of potassium to sodium of about 16:1. This is a stark difference to modern Western diets, in which this ratio is not only reduced, but actually contains more sodium than potassium.

Research and dietary recommendations tend to focus on reducing sodium intake. Because sodium (in the form of salt) is easy to come by, cheap, and abundant in prepared foods and fast food, this is undoubtedly good advice for most people, who consume far too much.

However, restoring a healthy potassium/sodium ratio by

also ensuring adequate potassium intake should be equally considered, as it's important for heart and bone health and reduces the risk of stroke and coronary heart disease. A large meta-analysis of RTCs and cohort studies provided high-quality evidence that increased potassium intake reduces blood pressure in people with hypertension and is associated with a significant (24%) lower risk of stroke.[15] Low potassium intakes have also been shown to be associated with increased arterial stiffness, a key risk factor for cardiovascular disease.[16] Meanwhile, another meta-analysis has shown higher potassium intakes to positively influence bone mineral density, a key marker of bone health.[17]

The reference nutrient intake of potassium for both male and female adults in the UK is 3,500mg. A detailed analysis of the UK National Diet and Nutrition Survey, a survey of food consumption and nutritional status across a large representative sample of people in the UK, showed that up to 23% of adults had inadequate intakes.[18] Meanwhile, in America, the National Health and Nutrition Examination Survey of nearly 10,000 adults showed that a staggering 97% didn't meet the recommended potassium intake (although the adequate intake in America is set higher, at 4,700mg).[19] Incidentally, 91% also consumed over the upper tolerable intake for sodium.

By comparison, studies show that vegans tend to have a significantly higher dietary intake of potassium than non-vegetarians. For example, in the Adventist Health Study, while all participants had a higher intake than the national US average (because a healthy diet is advocated for all Adventists), vegans still tended to have a potassium intake around 18% higher than non-vegetarians.[20] Vegans have this advantage when it comes to potassium intake because plant foods provide it in abundance. A selection of some of the best sources are listed in the table below.

FOOD	SERVING SIZE	TYPICAL POTASSIUM (mg)
Swiss chard, cooked	1 cup	961
Butter (lima) beans, cooked	1 cup	955
Baked potato, with skin	1 medium	926
Spinach, cooked	1 cup	839
Pinto beans, cooked	1 cup	746
Lentils, cooked	1 cup	731
Kidney beans, cooked	1 cup	717
Split peas, cooked	1 cup	710
Butternut squash, cooked	1 cup	582
Tomato juice	1 cup	556

(Data from USDA FoodData Central https://fdc.nal.usda.gov.)

It's interesting to note that although bananas do provide a good amount of potassium, with 422mg in a medium banana, there are many other foods that are much higher! I remember a distance cyclist I worked with years ago expressed concerns about having more than two bananas a day, because he'd heard from his coach that he could overdose on potassium – but the truth is you'd need eight bananas just to meet the daily requirements, and he could have even more if he wanted, as there's no set upper limit for potassium from foods.

• Magnesium

Magnesium is the fourth most abundant mineral in the human body and plays a vital role in general health as well as athletic performance, because of its involvement in energy metabolism, protein synthesis, creating and repairing DNA, muscle contractions, and regulating neurotransmitters. Research also suggests that magnesium deficiency could be a significant contributor to chronic, low-grade inflammation, which, as we've discussed, often underpins conditions such as high blood pressure, diabetes and cardiovascular disease.[21]

Most of the magnesium in the body is stored in the bones, where it plays a crucial role in the bone mineralization process. Magnesium in the bone can also act as a 'reservoir', to ensure that enough magnesium is made available to the body when needed, for instance when dietary intake is low. Suboptimal intake can therefore directly affect bone health, as demonstrated by studies showing that intake of magnesium (through both diet and supplementation) is strongly associated with markers of bone health.[22]

The reference nutrient intake for magnesium in adults in the UK is 300mg a day for men and 270mg a day for women. The UK National Diet and Nutrition Survey showed that average intakes are below this for all age groups, but notably averaging around 20% below the RNI for adults in their 20s and 15% below for adults in their 30s.[23]

Even marginal magnesium deficiency impairs exercise performance, and amplifies the oxidative stress resulting from strenuous exercise. Surveys show that intake of magnesium among athletes is often sub-optimal, especially in sports requiring weight control like wrestling or gymnastics.[24] This is another area where vegan athletes can have an advantage – studies show that vegans tend to have a higher magnesium intake than meat-eaters, for example 20% higher in a large UK cohort and 28% higher in the Adventist Health Study.[25, 26] That's because some of the best sources of magnesium include green leafy vegetables, legumes, nuts, seeds and whole grains – all typically higher in a healthy plant-based diet.

FOOD	SERVING SIZE	TYPICAL MAGNESIUM (mg)
Spinach, cooked	1 cup	157
Pumpkin seeds	28g	151
Chard, cooked	1 cup	150
Black beans, cooked	1 cup	120
Edamame beans, cooked	1 cup	99
Cashews, raw	28g	82
Chickpeas, cooked	1 cup	79
Almonds, raw	28g	75
Kidney beans, cooked	1 cup	74
Tofu, firm (calcium set)	½ cup	73

(Data from USDA FoodData Central https://fdc.nal.usda.gov.)

This is not an exhaustive list of nutrients that vegans tend to have an advantageous intake of – there are many other vitamins, antioxidants and other plant compounds which are naturally higher in a balanced plant-based diet, such as vitamins A, C, and K. This is one of the reasons I like to remind people of the bigger picture regarding plant-based nutrition, such as the powerful health benefits, performance advantages, and improved recovery. With that being said, there are some key nutrients for vegans, just as there are for every population, that are important to consider. In the next chapter we'll look at ways to optimize intake of these to further enhance any health and performance benefits, and help you thrive on your diet.

CHAPTER 5

KEY NUTRIENTS FOR VEGANS

We've seen that almost every population has key nutrients they ought to be mindful of, and while there are many significant health benefits to a plant-based diet, vegans are no exception and have some key nutrients too. Some of these may require supplementation or using fortified foods to meet your requirements, which is at least certainly the case for vitamin B_{12}. But with the vast majority of people using vitamin supplements anyway, I'd consider this a small price to pay to gain from all of the health benefits and potential improvements in performance.

You'll also see just how easy it is to incorporate all these nutrients into your diet. In fact, if you're eating a varied and balanced vegan diet, you're likely to be getting enough of most of these nutrients already. But, within this chapter, I hope you'll find lots of science-backed information to provide you with reassurance, and also some useful tips and tricks to make sure you're optimizing your nutrition, to see both immediate improvements in energy and vitality, as well as protecting your long-term health too.

There are no dietary reference values specifically set for athletes in the UK, and the reference nutrient intakes (RNIs) are broadly as recommended for the general population, which are designed to meet the needs of 97.5% of the population. In any case, the energy intake of the active person usually increases to match the energy requirements of physical activity, so a proportionate increase also occurs in micronutrient intake, often in amounts greatly exceeding RNIs.

Chapter 10 contains some of my favourite tried and tested recipes that incorporate these nutrients, to help you get as many of them naturally through your diet as possible. You'll see highlighted within the nutrition information of each recipe which ones are good sources of these key nutrients, so you can cross-reference back to this chapter to see how each nutrient is included.

Vitamin B12

For vegan athletes and non-athletes alike, considering your vitamin B_{12} intake is probably the most important message I'd like to convey in this book. I'm passionate about ensuring vegans get enough vitamin B_{12}, because almost every case of B_{12} deficiency is a wholly avoidable tragedy, and needlessly brings the health benefits of veganism into disrepute. So, if you only learn one lesson from this book, I hope that it's the information contained within these following paragraphs.

Vitamin B_{12} isn't produced by plants, so for vegans, and most vegetarians, it's the one vitamin which absolutely must be taken either in supplement form or by eating foods that are fortified with vitamin B_{12}. It's produced instead by microorganisms. In the case of meat, these microorganisms live in the stomach of the animals, and produce B_{12} which is absorbed into the bloodstream and accumulates in the animals' tissues. This is as long as the cattle graze on grass that has sufficient amounts of cobalt, a trace mineral that's required by those bacteria for B_{12} production. Non-grass-fed cattle (the vast majority), or those grazing in low-cobalt soils, are fed with B_{12} fortified feed. In the case of supplements, the bacteria are simply cultured without the need for an animal as a host, and produce B_{12} as part of a fermentation process.

Vitamin B_{12} plays a variety of important roles, ranging from DNA synthesis, red blood cell formation, and the formation of myelin – the protective sheath that surrounds nerve fibres. So, clinical signs of B_{12} deficiency can include fatigue and weakness due to low numbers of healthy red blood cells, as well as tingling, numbness, memory loss and confusion owing to nerve cell damage. If left unchecked over time, some of this neurological damage can be irreversible.

Along with folate, vitamin B_{12} is also crucial for the breakdown of homocysteine, a metabolite produced when certain proteins are broken down. Even slightly elevated levels of homocysteine are strongly associated with increased risk of cardiovascular disease, pregnancy complications, and several other chronic diseases.[1, 2] So, while it's common for most vegans to get enough B_{12} to avoid the overt clinical symptoms such as anaemia and nerve cell damage, it's also really important to ensure an adequate intake to avoid an increase in homocysteine, which can, without necessarily showing any obvious symptoms, increase risk of several chronic diseases.

Another thing to consider is that B_{12} is a water-soluble vitamin that can be stored in the liver for quite some time. So for some people first adopting a vegan diet without suitable supplementation or fortification, B_{12} stores can slowly decline without showing any symptoms for many months or even years. This has led some into a false sense of security, believing that they don't need B_{12}, meanwhile deficiency is slowly creeping up on them.

Studies usually show a higher prevalence of B_{12} deficiency among vegans and vegetarians. For example, a systematic review of 40 studies that assessed the B_{12} status of vegans and vegetarians in multiple countries from Europe, Africa, Asia, Australasia and North America, found that in general, B_{12} status was significantly lower in vegans than in omnivores. However, deficiency rates varied massively between populations. For example, in some areas, up to 86.5% of vegans had low B_{12} levels, while in the UK, a large cohort study showed that 52% of vegans were classed as vitamin B_{12} deficient.[3] But in populations which appropriately included B_{12} fortified foods in their diet, 0% had deficiencies.[4]

So B_{12} deficiency among vegans is totally avoidable. To me there is a lack of public health messaging regarding B_{12}, despite the growing popularity of plant-based diets. There has rightly been a big public health push in other areas, for example to encourage the use of vitamin D supplements for everyone in the UK, and I believe there should be an equally big drive for information around vitamin B_{12} among vegans, vegetarians and all over-50s (that's because a high proportion of older people may mal-absorb food-bound vitamin B_{12}, owing to the reduced absorption rate in the gut associated with ageing).

As we saw in Chapter 3, the best-quality studies we have show that vegan diets are associated with profound improvements in risk of numerous chronic diseases. This is despite the relatively high prevalence of vitamin B_{12} deficiency. So I can only imagine what further health improvements would be seen if *all* vegans supplemented appropriately to ensure a suitable B_{12} intake.

The reference nutrient intake for vitamin B_{12} in the UK is 1.5μg a day. However, some countries have set their reference intakes much higher: 2.4μg a day in the US, Canada, and Australia, and 4μg in most other European countries. If you're getting your vitamin B_{12} from fortified foods (see table below), it would be sensible therefore to aim for 4μg a day as per European guidelines or at least 3μg a day as endorsed by the Vegan Society.[5]

FORTIFIED FOOD SOURCE	SERVING SIZE	TYPICAL VITAMIN B12 (µg)
Fortified nutritional yeast*	5g	2.2
Marmite	8g	1.9
Fortified oat milk*	200ml	0.7
Fortified breakfast cereal*	40g	0.6
Fortified vegan spread*	10g	0.5
Fortified soy yoghurt*	120ml	0.4

(Data from USDA FoodData Central https://fdc.nal.usda.gov and individual brand nutrition information.)

* Amounts vary between brands and from country to country – please check the label.

You can see that it's relatively straightforward to reach 3–4μg of vitamin B_{12} a day by including a few portions of fortified foods, ideally spread throughout the day. Depending on your lifestyle, food preferences and accessibility, you may, however, prefer to take your vitamin B_{12} in supplement form. If this is the case, the daily recommendations change to either:

Taking a daily supplement providing at least 10μg

OR

Taking a weekly supplement providing at least 2000μg

This is because the less frequently you obtain B_{12}, the more you need to take, as it's absorbed better in small amounts. The recommendations above take this absorption rate into account and are advised by the British Dietetic Association.[6]

If you're an athlete, all the advantages of ensuring an adequate B_{12} intake are particularly important to you. The ability to produce sufficient healthy red blood cells to supply the muscles with oxygen during exercise is vital for peak performance, as is maintaining healthy nerve cells for motor skills. So if you weren't already, I sincerely hope this section has inspired you, now understanding the importance of ensuring an adequate B_{12} intake!

Iron

Most vegans will have been quizzed at some stage about their iron intake, and many sources will tell you that you need to take an iron supplement to achieve normal iron status. However, it's quite possible – in fact easy – for most vegans to maintain adequate iron stores naturally through the diet. We'll discuss here why iron is so important, and how to boost iron intake and absorption on a plant-based diet.

As with all minerals in our diet, iron is used in many ways in the body. It's needed to make new cells, hormones, neurotransmitters and amino acids, it helps many enzymes in the energy-generating pathways, and is also required for making new DNA. However, most iron in the body is found in two proteins: haemoglobin (found in red blood cells) and myoglobin (found in muscle cells). The iron in haemoglobin allows the red blood cells to carry oxygen from the lungs to the tissues – particularly muscle cells during exercise – in order for them to produce energy. Myoglobin holds and stores oxygen within our muscle cells, ready for use during exercise.

With insufficient iron intake, the production of haemoglobin is inhibited, and when its concentration in blood drops below the normal range, it's known as anaemia. This means your body's ability to transport oxygen for generating energy becomes impaired, and is felt as fatigue, tiredness and weakness. Anaemia can therefore be felt in everyday life, and as expected, can dramatically impair athletic performance.

Iron deficiency is the most commonly reported nutritional disorder in the world, and in the UK up to 40% of adult women have intakes below recommended levels.[7] The high prevalence of low iron intake is why all bread and flour produced in the UK must by law be fortified with iron. So this is a nutrient that's important for everyone to consider, not just vegans.

The reference intakes of iron for adults in the UK are 8.7mg a day, or 14.8mg a day for pre-menopausal women. The reason the reference intake is so much higher for women is to factor for the higher losses from monthly menstrual bleeding. Let's take a look at a selection of plant-based iron sources to see how straightforward it is to meet these intakes on a vegan diet:

FOOD	SERVING SIZE	TYPICAL IRON (mg)
Lentils cooked	1 cup	6.6
Spinach, cooked	1 cup	6.4
Tofu, firm	100g	5.4
Chickpeas, cooked	1 cup	4.7
Fortified breakfast cereals*	40g	2–6
Pumpkin seeds	30g	4.2
Kidney beans, cooked	1 cup	3.9
Quinoa, cooked	1 cup	2.8
Peas, cooked	1 cup	2.5
Cashews, raw	25g	2
Potato, skin on	1 medium	1.9
Oats, uncooked	½ cup	1.9
Bread, wholemeal	1 slice	0.9

(Data from USDA FoodData Central https://fdc.nal.usda.gov and individual brand nutrition information.)

* Amounts vary between brands and from country to country – please check the label.

It's clear how easy it is to ensure enough iron is consumed on a plant-based diet that's varied. A simple serving of curried chickpeas in a baked potato would provide 6.6mg of iron. Fortunately, many of the foods high in iron (such as lentils, beans, other pulses and nuts) are also high in protein, so by including plenty of these foods in your diet you're ensuring needs for both iron and protein are met.

Several studies, including a large UK cohort study, show that iron intake of vegans tends to in fact be higher than omnivores.[8] Importantly, however, iron stores in vegans are usually lower, despite this higher intake,[9] the reason being the differences in the iron form derived from plant and animal sources.

As discussed in Chapter 3, iron from plant sources comes in the form of non-haem iron, whereas meat contains haem iron. The lower iron status in vegans and vegetarians is thought to be because of the lower absorption of non-haem iron compared to haem iron, rather than lower absolute intake. So it's important to include a variety of iron-rich foods, but also to ensure that the iron you consume is well absorbed. To do that, you just need to understand the dietary factors that can either inhibit iron absorption or enhance it.

Of the dietary factors that can enhance iron absorption, vitamin C seems to be the most powerful. Incorporating just 25–75mg of vitamin C (equivalent to one small orange or half a cup of cooked broccoli) is enough to boost the iron absorption by three to four times.[10] Other organic acids can help with iron absorption too, for example, acetic acids in vinegars, lactic acid in fermented foods, and other organic acids found in many fruits like malic acid, tartaric acid and citric acid. These other organic acids can increase iron absorption, although not quite to the extent of vitamin C.[11]

On the other hand, there are several dietary factors that can inhibit the absorption of non-haem iron, the main ones being tea and coffee – the tannins and other polyphenols within them, including decaffeinated and some herbal teas, are packed with antioxidants and are very healthy, but can significantly reduce the amount of plant-based iron we consume from being absorbed. So if you're a tea or coffee drinker, it could significantly help with iron absorption if you aim to have them between meals rather than with (or soon after) your food.

Another inhibitory factor is the phytate contained in seeds, grains, legumes and nuts. All these foods are forms of plant seeds, and contain phytates to act as the main storage form of phosphorus, which is released and used for growth by the plant when the seeds germinate. These phytates can inhibit the absorption of iron (as well as some other minerals like zinc and calcium). Because of this, some people dub phytates with the term 'anti-nutrient', which I find particularly unhelpful because it puts some people off eating grains, legumes, nuts and seeds, which is a travesty because they all have proven powerful health benefits. The reality is, phytates are a good example of a nutrient that can have both helpful and unhelpful qualities, depending on circumstances. On the one hand, they're potent antioxidants, and some scientists suggest they could be part of the reason why whole grains are linked to lower risk of colon cancer.[12, 13] On the other hand, they can inhibit the absorption of some minerals. Luckily, many of the natural processes that already happen to foods, like leavening bread, soaking and cooking beans, and fermenting soy products, reduce the inhibitory effect of the phytates.

Also vitamin C can counteract these inhibitory effects,[14] so I encourage my clients not to worry too much about phytates. The key message here is to instead focus on incorporating plenty of vitamin C and other organic acids into your meals, alongside lots of iron-rich plant foods. For example, try including fresh lemon juice in your salad dressing, adding some vitamin C-rich vegetables like broccoli and red peppers into your stir-fries, or making smoothies that contain iron-rich leafy greens combined with vitamin C-rich berries. At the same time, aiming to drink any tea or coffee between meals instead of with meals will help too.

Fun fact: vegans often have higher iron levels than vegetarians, because cheese and eggs which are frequently included as the protein group in meals contain very little iron. Instead, vegans tend to eat more beans, pulses and tofu in plant-based dishes, all of which are packed with iron!

Zinc

Zinc is an essential mineral that's required for the activity of over 300 enzymes involved in most major metabolic pathways. So it plays important roles in immune function, protein synthesis, wound healing, and DNA synthesis. Several of the enzymes that zinc plays a role in are also vital for energy metabolism, and so are critical for sports performance.

A systematic review and meta-analysis of zinc status in vegetarians and vegans showed that those following a plant-based diet had dietary zinc intakes and serum zinc concentrations that were significantly lower than those of non-vegetarians.[15] Studies also show that many athletes, whether vegan or not, have sub-optimal zinc intakes – especially those who restrict calorie intake to meet weight goals, and some endurance athletes who require high intakes of carbohydrates at the expense of other food groups to fuel their training and events.[16] However, with a little planning and perhaps a few simple dietary tweaks, it should be easy for most vegans to meet their zinc requirements naturally from the diet and without the use of supplementation.

The UK dietary reference values of zinc for adults in the UK are 7mg a day for women and 9.5mg a day for men.

FOOD	SERVING SIZE	TYPICAL ZINC (mg)
Nutrition yeast flakes*	5g	6
Baked beans, tinned	1 cup	3.5
Oats, uncooked	1 cup	3.2
Lentils, cooked	1 cup	2.5
Spring greens, cooked	1 cup	2.5
Chickpeas, cooked	1 cup	2.5
Pumpkin seeds	28g	2.1
Quinoa, cooked	1 cup	2.0
Black beans, cooked	1 cup	1.9
Peas, cooked	1 cup	1.9
Kidney beans, cooked	1 cup	1.8
Tofu, firm*	100g	1.6
Cashews, raw	25g	1.6
Spinach, cooked	1 cup	1.4
Brown rice, cooked	1 cup	1.2

(Data from USDA FoodData Central https://fdc.nal.usda.gov and individual brand nutrition information.)

* Amounts vary between brands and from country to country – please check the label.

Looking at this table, you can see that it's pretty easy to meet your requirements of zinc by following a balanced, varied diet consisting of plenty of pulses, grains, vegetables, nuts and seeds. However, like iron, it's useful to think about the absorption of zinc as well as the overall intake. That's because phytates, intakes of which tend to be higher in a vegan diet, can bind with zinc and inhibit its absorption. For this reason, some sources like the US Institute of Medicine recommend that vegans aim for higher amounts than the daily reference intake.[17]

The advice here is somewhat similar to promoting iron absorption: leavening bread (e.g. most risen breads rather than flatbreads), soaking and cooking beans, grains and seeds, and fermenting soy products, all reduce the inhibitory effect of the phytates.

An equally effective and perhaps more practical way to enhance zinc absorption is, again just like improving iron absorption, consuming organic acids (rich in most fresh fruits and fermented foods like sourdough bread and tempeh) to reduce the binding of zinc by the phytates and therefore increase its absorbability. So if you're already following this advice for enhancing iron absorption, this will help with zinc absorption too. Try smoothies containing zinc-rich greens along with berries, topping porridge oats with fresh fruit, incorporating fruit into salads or dressings, or having fresh fruit for dessert after a meal.

Both onion and garlic have also been shown to significantly improve the bioavailability of zinc and iron from grains and pulses.[18] Luckily, meals like soups, stews and curries, including many in the recipes included in Chapter 10, contain onion and garlic alongside zinc-rich pulses and vegetables. So, to ensure you maintain adequate zinc levels, you should strive to meet or exceed the daily reference intakes, and include other methods of improving absorption such as incorporating fermented foods, eating plenty of fresh fruit, and using onion and garlic in your cooking alongside plenty of zinc-rich plant-foods.

Omega-3 fatty acids

Many people find dietary fats very confusing, and it's one of the areas where there are extremes of advice, especially if you search online. Here, we'll break down the science into simple take-away messages and actionable advice, based on the best available evidence, to make sure you're optimizing your fat intake and incorporating plenty of healthy unsaturated fats, particularly omega-3 fatty acids, into your diet.

There are many classes of dietary fats. In general, it's advised to keep intake of saturated and trans fats to a minimum, while mono- and polyunsaturated fats have been associated with health benefits when consumed in moderation and as part of a varied diet. Remember from Chapter 3, minimizing saturated fat intake is one of the key mechanisms by which a plant-based diet reaps such potent health benefits.

Also bear in mind that all dietary fat sources contain a variety of fats in differing proportions. For example, many people think of salmon when talking about omega-3, but salmon also contains omega-6, monounsaturated fat, and saturated fat. Likewise, although olive oil is often described as an unsaturated fat because it's high in monounsaturated fats (with a little omega-3 and some omega-6), it also contains some saturated fat.

The body is capable of synthesizing most of the fatty acids it needs from food. But there are two considered 'essential' because our bodies can't make them and they're critical for health. These are linoleic acid (LA, an omega-6 fatty acid) and alpha-linoleic acid (ALA, an omega-3 fatty acid). They're both used to create a family of important signalling molecules known as eicosanoids, which are used for many functions within the body such as regulating cell growth and controlling blood pressure. But, perhaps most notably, they also help to control inflammation and the immune response. The eicosanoids created from omega-3 fats reduce the inflammation response, while those created from omega-6 fats encourage inflammation. We'll discuss the role of inflammation further in Chapter 6, but put simply, although acute inflammation can be useful to protect your body from infection or injury, long-term low-level inflammation is associated with a variety of ailments ranging from arthritis to asthma.

During human evolution, it's estimated that the ratio of omega-6 to omega-3 in the diet was around 1:1. Nowadays, in the West, diets are particularly high in omega-6, and tend to be low in omega-3, so much so that the ratio is on average more like 16:1.[19] That's because so many of the foods we eat are made with vegetable oils, such as most deep-fried foods, fast foods, crisps, chips, and many processed foods like cakes, biscuits and cookies. As you can see from the table opposite, some of the most common vegetable oils used for frying and in processed foods (sunflower, safflower, corn oils) are extremely high in omega-6.

There's no 'magic' omega-6:3 ratio we should aim for. Also, it would be extremely laborious to calculate the ratios precisely, particularly because most foods contain a variety of different fats in varying proportions. Still, studies show that a much lower ratio than is commonplace in the West can have significant health benefits: a ratio of 2.5:1 reduced cell proliferation in patients with colorectal cancer; a ratio of 3:1 suppressed inflammation in patients with rheumatoid arthritis; and a ratio of 5:1 had beneficial effects on patients with asthma, while a ratio of 10:1 seemed to make the condition worse.[20] So it seems that keeping that ratio as low as possible could decrease inflammation and the risk of several inflammation-associated diseases.

In practical terms, to improve your omega-6:3 ratio, it would be prudent to strive to include 1–2 servings per day of the plant foods that supply omega-3 fats, such as 1 tablespoon of ground flaxseed, chia seeds, hemp seeds, 1 teaspoon of their oils, or 28g of walnuts. Other plant sources of omega-3 are found in the table below. Meanwhile, try to moderate the amount of omega-6 in the diet by limiting foods cooked in sunflower, safflower and corn oils (including most fast foods!).

	FOOD	PORTION	OMEGA-6	OMEGA-3	OMEGA-6:3 RATIO
Foods with favourable omega 6:3 ratios	Flaxseed	1 Tbsp	0.5g	2.1g	1:4
	Flaxseed oil	1 tsp	0.6g	2.4g	1:4
	Chia seeds	1 Tbsp	0.9g	2.6g	1:3
	Hemp seed oil	1 tsp	0.8g	2.3g	1:3
	Cold-pressed rapeseed oil	1 tsp	0.9g	0.4g	2:1
	Hemp seeds	1 Tbsp	2.8g	0.9g	3:1
	Walnuts	14 halves (28g)	10.8g	2.6g	4:1
	Edamame beans	1 cup	2.7g	0.6g	5:1
Cooking fats with unfavourable omega 6:3 ratio	Corn oil	1 Tbsp	7.2g	0.2g	36:1
	Sunflower oil	1 Tbsp	3.9g	<0.1g	>40:1
	Cottonseed oil	1 Tbsp	7.0g	<0.1g	>70:1
	Safflower oil	1 Tbsp	10.1g	<0.1g	>100:1

(Data from USDA FoodData Central https://fdc.nal.usda.gov and individual brand nutrition information.)

Top Tip: Grinding your flaxseeds (or buying them ready-ground) will greatly increase the absorption of omega-3 and other nutrients. If storing ground flaxseeds, keep them in the fridge, as the fats can begin to oxidize over time as room temperature (the same goes for walnuts too, once the bag is opened).

Other healthy fat sources include other nuts (e.g. peanuts, cashews, almonds and their nut butters), seeds (e.g. sesame, sunflower and pumpkin seeds), avocado, and extra virgin olive oil in moderation. None of these have much omega-3 but they're made up primarily of monounsaturated fats, so won't impact your omega-3:6 ratio nearly as much as cooking oils like sunflower or vegetable oil. Nuts, seeds and avocados also have countless other important nutrients including fibre, protein and phytochemicals, so including them in your diet brings important benefits.

As well as the ALA omega-3 from the sources above, there are two other important omega-3 fatty acids to consider that are also important for health – EPA and DHA. These are commonly found in oily fish and are long-chain omega-3 fatty acids, whereas ALA from plant sources is a short-chain omega-3 fatty acid. Our bodies can take the ALA from plant foods and elongate it to the long-chain omega-3s, EPA and DHA. But that conversion rate can be limiting, and differs from person to person and between sexes (women tend to convert ALA to EPA and DHA a little more efficiently).[21] See the diagram opposite, which shows how the long-chain omega-3s can be produced from dietary ALA, as well as obtained directly from food.

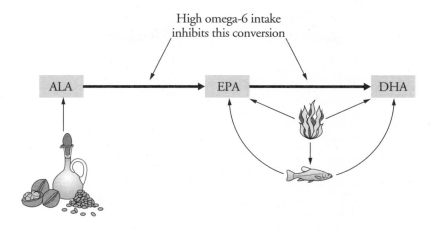

Because vegans and vegetarians don't eat fish, in the UK they've been shown to have lower blood levels of these long-chain fatty acids.[22] One method to improve the efficiency of this conversion is by limiting omega-6 intake: a diet high in omega-6 creates competition for the enzymes that desaturate and elongate ALA omega-3 to EPA and DHA.[23] This is another reason why limiting intake of omega-6 rich cooking oils and fried foods can be beneficial.

In the UK, there is no specific recommendation for a dose of omega-3. However, in many other countries, daily reference intakes have been set. For example, in the US and Canada the daily reference intake has been set for ALA at 1.1g/day for women and 1.6g/day for men, and the European Food Safety Authority and World Health Organization recommend getting 0.5% of your energy from ALA. Vegans may be at an advantage here, because consumption of nuts and seeds, including those highest in ALA, tends to be higher.

In the US and Canada, there are no reference values for EPA and DHA because ALA is the only omega-3 that's considered essential. However, in the UK, the Eatwell Guide recommends eating one portion of oily fish a week in order to obtain the long-chain omega-3s, and the European Food Safety Authority recommends a more specific daily intake of 250mg of EPA+DHA.[24, 25]

If you wanted to consume long-chain EPA and DHA omega-3 fats directly, rather than relying on your body creating them from the ALA in your diet, there is a vegan alternative to eating fish or fish oils: algae. In fact, fish don't make EPA and DHA themselves – they get it from the algae they eat (or small crustaceans that eat the algae). So you too could get it directly from the source and cut out the 'middleman' and get long-chain omega-3 from algal oil supplements. Another advantage of getting EPA and DHA from algal oil supplements rather than fish consumption is that algae grown for supplements are grown and harvested in contamination-free tanks. Meanwhile, because we've polluted our oceans, seafood and even purified fish oils contain pollutants like PCBs, dioxins and heavy metals.[26, 27] Although the research into algal oil supplementation is relatively young, it shows that it helps raise omega-3 blood levels as effectively as fish, could help reduce risk of CVD and could reduce inflammation, all without those pollutants and the gastrointestinal complaints often associated with fish oils, such as highly embarrassing fishy odorous belches.[28–31]

The evidence for omega-3 supplementation for athletes is fairly limited. Because omega-3 has the potential to reduce inflammation, it's thought that it might improve muscle soreness after exercise and potentially increase muscle mass and strength while training.[32] But meta-analyses of trials in humans haven't shown consistent results, although it's relatively early days in the research, so this may change.[33, 34]

So it's really down to personal choice whether or not you

choose to supplement with algae-derived EPA and DHA. If you are prone to inflammatory injuries, you could give it a try and see if you notice any improvements. Even if bumping up your omega-3 intake has no effect on any nagging injuries or muscle soreness, it could still provide other health benefits. Either way, it's still always a good idea to incorporate plenty of the plant-based sources of omega-3 and try to limit intake of fried and processed foods in order to moderate omega-6 intake.

Calcium

Calcium plays important roles in a wide variety of bodily functions, ranging from intracellular messaging and blood clotting, to neurological function and muscular contractions. And of course, as many of us are taught from a young age, it's vital for bone health. In fact, 99% of calcium in our bodies is found in the bones (approximately 1.2kg in the average adult) and it's the most abundant mineral in the body.

It's useful to remember that bone is a living tissue. It's constantly being broken down and rebuilt, replacing existing bone structure with new bone structure in a process known as bone turnover. In fact, the adult skeleton is remodelled and replaced approximately every 10 years. It's staggering to think that your skeleton now is almost completely distinct from your skeleton 10 years ago!

An adequate intake of calcium is important for this bone turnover process, keeping bones healthy and strong. It's also vital for reaching a healthy peak bone mass, which is the point at which bones reach their maximum strength and density. As you can see in the graph on page 92, this usually occurs in the early 20s in women and late 20s in men. From this age, bone mass usually stays roughly the same for about

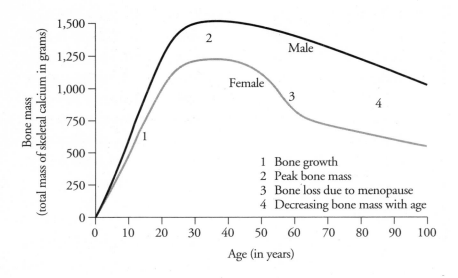

10–15 years, before slowly declining with age (with an accel-erated loss for women during menopause). Diets with insuf-ficient amounts of calcium during growth can lead to a lower peak bone mass, and a deficiency in adulthood can result in faster rate of loss with age. This can have implications for bone health, increasing risk of stress fractures in athletes,[35] and of osteoporosis in later life.

However, when people think about the nutrition and life-style factors that affect bone health, most think solely of cal-cium. Of course, calcium is critical, but the reality is that there are many other important factors that can significantly influence it too. Other nutrients that are vital for bone health include magnesium and potassium, both of which, you may remember from Chapter 4, tend to be higher in vegans. There are several other vitamins and minerals needed for metabolic processes related to bone, including manganese, phosphorus, copper, iron, zinc, vitamins A, C, K, and the B vitamins, all of which are supplied in ample amounts in a healthy, balanced vegan diet. Weight-bearing exercise and keeping a healthy weight can also positively affect bone health, while smoking, alcohol, excessive caffeine and high salt intakes can be detrimental.[36]

Interestingly, if you look at countries' dairy intake and risk of bone fracture (a good population-level indicator of bone health), countries that consume more dairy have higher risk of fractures[37] (see the graph below). This is an interesting concept, but think back to Chapter 2 – this type of evidence

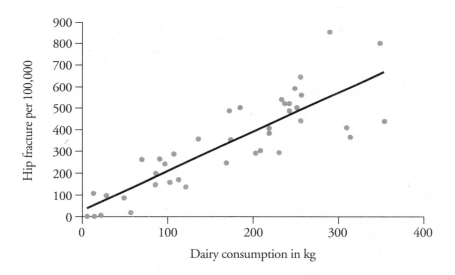

is cross-sectional and so can't prove causality or rule out other confounding factors. For example, countries consuming the most dairy tend to be more affluent, with higher proportions of people working in sedentary, indoor jobs, and rates of obesity tend to be higher, both of which can also affect bone health. Nonetheless, this data is interesting and shows that consuming more dairy certainly isn't a surefire way of protecting your bone health.

The reason calcium is a key nutrient for vegans is because most people in the West get a significant amount of their calcium (around 40%) from cow's milk and other dairy products.[38] So it's perhaps no surprise that most studies show that calcium intake in vegans tends to be lower than in vegetarians and omnivores.[39] And this translates into practical implications: a recent meta-analysis of 20 studies with a total of 37,000 participants showed that vegans tended to have lower bone mineral density and slightly higher risk of bone fracture.[40] This was also found in a large UK cohort study following 34,000 people over five years: a higher fracture risk among vegans vs vegetarians and omnivores.[41] However, importantly, in this study the researchers also statistically adjusted for calcium intake, and found that among vegans who consumed just 525mg/day or more of calcium, bone fracture risk wasn't increased.

So it's certainly not the case for all vegans, and it's the purpose of this section to make sure you fall into the category of vegans who consume enough calcium to keep your bones just as healthy as those of omnivores. In fact, because a vegan diet tends to be higher in other important minerals like magnesium and potassium, and vegans are more likely to be a healthy weight, it's quite possible with adequate intake of calcium (and vitamin D, covered in the next section) for you to have healthier bones than non-vegans. And you'll also see that it's very easy to do, with some basic planning.

The dietary reference value of calcium for adults in the UK is 700mg a day for both men and women (with higher requirements during growth, pregnancy and breastfeeding). Let's take a look at the calcium content of a selection of plant-based foods to see how we can reach that intake:

FOOD	SERVING SIZE	TYPICAL CALCIUM (mg)
Tofu, firm, calcium-set*	120g	420
Fortified nut, oat, rice, or soy milk*	200ml glass	240
Pak choy, cooked	1 cup	158
Fortified soy yoghurt*	120g pot	150
Spring greens, cooked	1 cup	143
Dried figs	80g	130
Tahini	2 Tbsp	130
Tempeh, cooked	120g	115
Edamame beans, cooked	1 cup	98
Curly kale, cooked	1 cup	90
Chickpeas, cooked	1 cup	80
Cabbage, cooked	1 cup	72
Almonds, raw	28g	70
Broccoli, cooked	1 cup	62
Brussels sprouts, cooked	1 cup	56

(Data from USDA FoodData Central https://fdc.nal.usda.gov and the UK Composition of Foods Dataset https://www.gov.uk/government/publications/composition-of-foods-integrated-dataset-cofid and individual brand nutrition information.)

* Amounts vary between brands and from country to country – please check the label.

You can see that plenty of plant foods contain lots of calcium. But, as well as getting plenty of calcium in the diet, we should also think about the absorbability. While humans absorb about 30% of the calcium in cow's milk, we can absorb up to 60% of the calcium in some vegetables, making them a fantastic source of calcium. The key is incorporating vegetables that are low in compounds called oxalates, which can bind to calcium in the gut and inhibit how much is absorbed. Low-oxalate vegetables include most of the Brassica family of vegetables, such as those listed in the table on page 95 (pak choy, spring greens, kale, broccoli, Brussels sprouts and cabbage). These vegetables have the magical combination of a high calcium content along with low levels of oxalates, which means lots of highly absorbable calcium.

On the other hand, some vegetables might at first appear to be great sources of calcium, owing to their high calcium content, but they also have high levels of oxalates, meaning that much less is absorbed. For example, cooked spinach has around 245mg of calcium per cup, but due to its high levels of oxalates, only around 5% is absorbed. Other high-oxalate vegetables include Swiss chard, rhubarb and beetroot. Of course, that doesn't mean you should avoid these foods, as they're highly nutritious and provide many profound health benefits – you just shouldn't rely on them for your calcium intake.

In terms of other vegan sources, the amount of calcium from fortified vegan milks, most legumes, nuts and seeds tends to be a little less well absorbed, but still provides a useful contribution, with absorption rates of these foods ranging from roughly 17–24%.[42] So a diet consisting of a wide variety of plant foods, including lots of leafy greens (especially from the Brassica family) alongside pulses, nuts and seeds, can easily meet the daily reference intake levels. This is made even easier with the addition of fortified foods such as tofu (that's set using calcium), plant milks, yoghurts and cereals.

Does meat 'leach' calcium from your bones?

I have an admission to make – I used to take a little satisfaction in telling people that eating a lot of meat can weaken our bones. The theory was that because a high meat diet acidifies the body (due to the high level of sulphur-containing amino acids in meat), calcium was taken from our bones to neutralize that acidity. This theory was based on numerous studies showing that adding meat to the diet resulted in more calcium being lost in the urine.[43] But the most recent and robust science has disproved that theory. Scientists, using a method called stable isotopes, are able to 'tag' calcium fed to participants. It turns out that the extra calcium in the urine when eating a high protein diet was that same 'tagged' calcium, so those increased urinary losses seem to come from the calcium we eat, not from our bones. [44-46] This is because protein can boost the absorption of calcium, which is then filtered through our kidneys and excreted in the urine.

So there may be numerous other detrimental effects of a high meat diet, and we know we don't need meat or dairy to have extremely healthy bones, but if we're to go on the best available evidence, we can no longer say that the acidity of meat weakens our bones.

Vitamin D

We've covered calcium in some detail, especially regarding its relationship with bone health. But, as discussed, there are many other important factors and nutrients that are also vital for bone health. A key one is vitamin D, which our body needs to maintain blood calcium levels.[47] As with all nutrients, however, vitamin D has numerous roles within the body. For example, it's involved in the modulation of cell growth, neuromuscular and immune function, and reduction of inflammation. So it's vital to make sure we get enough vitamin D.

It's often referred to as the 'sunshine vitamin', because vitamin D can be made in the skin when it's exposed to sunlight – specifically ultraviolet B (UVB) rays. In the skin, those UVB rays convert a form of cholesterol found in the membrane of skin cells into vitamin D_3. From here, vitamin D_3 goes through a series of conversions in the liver, then the kidneys, to calcitriol – its hormonally active form, whose main function is to control blood calcium levels. A key way in which it does this is by promoting calcium (and phosphate) absorption from the intestine: when there is a vitamin D deficiency, absorption of calcium in the intestines can be over 50% less efficient (10–15% of dietary calcium absorption vs around 30% absorption when vitamin D is sufficient).[48]

It's very difficult to know exactly how much vitamin D is synthesized from sun exposure because of the number, and complexity, of factors that affect the synthesis of vitamin D by the skin. For instance, skin colour can impact vitamin D synthesis – people with dark skin, such as those from African, Afro-Caribbean or South Asian backgrounds, may require more sun exposure to synthesize vitamin D, as higher melanin concentration in the skin absorbs some of the UVB rays. Likewise, people with very fair skin may require sunblock, which limits the skin's exposure to UVB rays. Other factors can affect sun exposure too, for instance office workers who spend most of the time inside, those who cover their skin for religious reasons, or institutionalized people such as those in care homes or hospitals who may not be able to get outdoors as much.

Although there is some evidence to suggest vegans and vegetarians may be at a higher risk of vitamin D deficiency, factors such as sun exposure, skin colour and supplementation have been shown to be much more important predictors of vitamin D status than intake from food sources.[49, 50] This is evident in the seasonal variability in serum vitamin D levels in the UK: the National Diet and Nutrition Survey (NDNS) showed that 8% of adults had low vitamin D levels in the summer, which increased to a staggering two out of five people – 39% – in the winter months.[51]

For athletes, this is of particular importance, because low vitamin D status has been associated with increased risk of stress fractures.[52] The military is a very physically active group that's been studied a lot, and a meta-analysis showed an association between vitamin D status and risk of stress fractures in military personnel.[53] However, an interesting pilot study in collegiate athletes has shown that regular supplementation significantly reduces risk of stress fractures.[54]

There were no specific recommendations for vitamin D intake in the UK for the general population until relatively recently: in 2016 the Scientific Advisory Committee on Nutrition (SACN) updated its advice and now suggests that everyone in the UK (aged over 1 year) get 10μg (400 iu) of vitamin D a day. Since it's difficult for people to meet this recommendation from dietary sources, the SACN suggests **everyone** in the UK considers taking a daily supplement, especially during the autumn and winter months.[55]

Vitamin D is listed in this section as a key nutrient for

vegans because there are hardly any vegan dietary sources, with the exception of certain mushrooms (such as shiitake) that have been exposed to UV light (either sunlight or some that are exposed to artificial UV lighting). So it may be of particular importance for vegans to follow the government-backed advice for everyone to consider a daily supplement or eat vitamin D-fortified foods, especially in the autumn and winter months, and even in the summer months if you do not get regular safe sun exposure or have darker skin. Here are some tips from the NHS about how to safely get vitamin D from sunlight:[56]

- In the UK, most people can make enough vitamin D from being out in the sun daily for short periods with their forearms, hands or lower legs uncovered and without sunscreen from late March or early April to the end of September, especially from 11 a.m. to 3 p.m.
- It's not known exactly how much time is needed in the sun to make enough vitamin D to meet the body's requirements. This is because there are a number of factors that can affect how vitamin D is made, such as your skin colour and how much skin you have exposed (longer periods of exposure may be needed for those with darker skin).
- Be aware that prolonged exposure (for example, leading to burning or tanning) is unlikely to provide additional benefit.[57]
- The longer you stay in the sun, especially for prolonged periods without sun protection, the greater your risk of skin cancer.

- If you plan to be out in the sun for long, cover up with suitable clothing, sunglasses, seeking shade and applying at least SPF15 sunscreen.

Two notes on supplements

1. There are two types of vitamin D supplement: D_2 and D_3. Both can help you meet your vitamin D requirements, but it's been shown that D_3 is more efficient at raising blood vitamin D levels.[58] So vitamin D_3 supplements may be preferable.

2. With that being said, you may wish to find vitamin D_3 supplements certified as vegan, because the vitamin D used for many supplements and in many fortified foods is of animal origin, often made from lanolin (a waxy substance taken from sheep's wool). Vegan vitamin D_3 supplements are available that are derived from lichen (a fungi/algae-like organism).

Iodine

Iodine is an essential trace element, meaning you need it in very small amounts. Its main use in the body is as a component of thyroid hormones, made by the thyroid gland located at the front of the neck, and these hormones influence the metabolism of your body's cells. In other words, it regulates the speed at which your cells and tissues work. The thyroid hormones also regulate protein synthesis and enzymatic activity, and are important for brain and neurological development.

With an insufficient iodine intake, your thyroid gland is

unable to produce enough of these thyroid hormones, a condition known as hypothyroidism. As these hormones regulate metabolism, the cells and organs of your body can slow down. For example, your heart rate may become slower than normal, or your intestines may work sluggishly, leading to constipation. Other symptoms can include tiredness, feeling cold, weight gain, poor concentration and depression. Clearly, all these symptoms can significantly affect exercise performance. When you consider that athletes lose some iodine through heavy sweating during vigorous exercise or training in hot, humid conditions, you can see why it's an important nutrient not only for vegans, but for athletes too.[59]

Iodine deficiency affects around 2 billion people worldwide, with around 50 million of those presenting with clinical manifestations.[60] Thankfully, many countries have adopted a mandatory salt iodization policy (fortifying all table salt with iodine), which has seen the number of countries where iodine deficiency is a public health problem halve over the last decade.[61]

Still, the UK is one of the few European countries without regulations on salt iodization, and iodine deficiency is prevalent. The National Diet and Nutrition Survey (NDNS) showed that low intake is common in some UK populations – for example 26% of girls aged 11–18 years had intakes below the lower reference range. They also monitor urinary iodine concentration, which showed that 46% of adults had urinary iodine levels below 100μg/L, which is indicative of mild deficiency.[62] So iodine deficiency is a nationwide issue, not just for vegans.

In the West, many people get the majority of their iodine from cow's milk and white fish, so it is a key nutrient for vegans – some studies show that vegans are more likely to have low iodine intakes and higher risk of iodine deficiency.[63]

In the UK, the daily reference intake is 140μg a day for both adult men and women, and athletes should aim to reach at least this level, because of the additional losses through sweat. So, let's take a look at the food sources of iodine to see how you can make sure you're getting enough.

FOOD	SERVING SIZE	TYPICAL IODINE (μg)
Iodine-fortified plant milk*	1 cup	53
Dried nori seaweed flakes	3g	44
Iodized salt*	¼ tsp	30
Most nuts	25g	5
Bread	1 slice	5
Most other vegetables	80g	3
Dried wakame seaweed	3g	505
Dried kombu/kelp seaweed	3g	13,220

(Data from the UK Composition of Foods Dataset, https://www.gov.uk/ government/publications/composition-of-foods-integrated-dataset-cofid and British Dietetic Association, https://www.bda.uk.com/resource/iodine.html and individual brand information.)

* Varies by brand.

The difficulty with estimating iodine intake from plant foods is that the iodine content can vary so much, depending on the iodine levels in the soil they're grown in. For example, crops grown near coastal areas tend to have higher iodine content,[64] while mountainous regions and river valleys prone to flooding usually have a lower content.[65] So while fruit, vegetables, grains and pulses might contribute towards your iodine intake a little, we shouldn't assume that they're reliable sources and we should consider some alternatives:

1. **Sea vegetables**. Seaweed is a more concentrated source of iodine which can be incorporated into the diet. For instance, topping salads, stews and stir-fries with dried nori seaweed flakes, or making vegan sushi with nori sheets, are delicious and simple ways to top up iodine intake. However, please bear in mind that some seaweeds (especially brown seaweeds like kelp, shown at the bottom of the table on page 103) can contain extremely high amounts of iodine, which can be toxic. For this reason, the British Dietetic Association don't recommend eating seaweed more than once a week.[66]

2. **Iodized salt.** The mandatory iodization of table salt in many countries has seen dramatic progress in the reduction of iodine deficiency disorders globally. However, using iodized salt comes with a **very important caveat**: do not let it encourage you to use more salt than you normally would. Even if your salt contains iodine, for most people it's still much healthier to limit salt intake (with the exception of athletes who sweat heavily, who may require more). Simply use a little iodized salt in place of regular salt in your cooking.

3. **Fortified foods.** Some foods now come fortified with iodine. For example, some plant milks contain over 50μg per cup, which can contribute significantly towards your intake.

4. **Supplements.** For most people, eating a variety of plant foods, eating some seaweed from time to

time, using a little iodized salt in your cooking, and perhaps incorporating some fortified foods should provide plenty of iodine. However, a supplement may be more appropriate for some people (e.g. if you don't like the taste of seaweed, or have been prescribed a low salt diet because of a medical condition). If so, look for a daily supplement that contains no more than 140µg. The British Dietetic Association recommends choosing a supplement in the form of potassium iodide or potassium iodate, because the amount of iodine in seaweed or kelp supplements can vary considerably from the value on the label and can provide excessive amounts of iodine.[67]

Why cow's milk is high in iodine

Did you know that goitre (extreme iodine deficiency, where the thyroid gland swells up) was endemic in the UK up until the early 1900s – in some areas, visible goitres were present in up to 50% of adults. But its eradication was completely unplanned and accidental: at the same time, farmers began to enrich cattle feed with iodine to improve the reproductive performance of livestock, which saw a spectacular rise in the iodine content of cow's milk (particularly in winter, when reliance on cattle feed is much higher). The introduction of iodine-based disinfectants used to clean cows' teats also contributed to the iodine content of the milk.[68] Simultaneously, successive governments put into effect policies to encourage the consumption of milk, mainly for economic reasons.[69] So the iodine content of cow's milk dramatically increased, and overall consumption of that milk nearly doubled, which made goitre a thing of the past. So if you decide to use fortified foods, iodized salt, or supplements to top up your iodine intake, it's a much more direct route than drinking milk from cows that are themselves fed with iodine supplements!

Selenium

Selenium is another essential trace element – so it's also only needed in very small amounts, but it's vital for several important processes in the body and must be obtained through the diet. Along with iodine, selenium is also required for the synthesis of thyroid hormones, and it's used to form a group of important proteins, known as seleno-proteins, which play a crucial role in protecting cells against free radical damage – which, as discussed in Chapter 3, can affect almost every cell and tissue in the body and can impact performance and recovery.

Not surprising, then, that there are many studies linking selenium status with potent health effects. On the one side, studies show that low selenium status is associated with increased mortality risk,[70] thyroid disorders,[71] inflammation, and immune-related diseases.[72] Other studies show that higher selenium content has some potential advantages, including reduced risk of breast, lung, oesophageal, gastric and prostate cancers,[73, 74] cardiovascular disease[75] and diabetes.[76] However, most of these studies show that a too high selenium status can also be damaging to health, suggesting that supplementation may only grant advantage if the nutrient is deficient to begin with. That's because although selenium is needed in small amounts for health, in higher doses it can be toxic.

This is why the daily reference intake in the UK is set at just 75μg a day for adult men and 60μg a day for adult women, and a safe upper limit has been set at 450μg a day by the Food Standards Agency.[77] Intakes above this level can have adverse effects on health. In fact in some of the studies mentioned above, adverse health effects were seen at intakes above just 200μg a day (over a prolonged period). So it's definitely important to get enough, but equally important not to overdo it.

In the UK, it's estimated that 39% of adults have selenium intakes below the lower reference intake (40μg a day).[78] So it's clear that this is a key nutrient for everyone, not just vegans. However, because many people in the West get much of their selenium from meat, fish, dairy and eggs, it's another nutrient that can be of particular importance for vegans – several studies show that vegans and vegetarians tend to have lower intakes of selenium than the general population.[79] That being said, it's easy to get enough selenium on a plant-based diet. Let's take a look at some plant-based sources:

FOOD	SERVING SIZE	TYPICAL SELENIUM (μg)
Brazil nuts	25g	40–1,100
Lentils (brown and green), cooked	1 cup	36
Pasta, cooked	1 cup	22
White mushrooms, raw	100g	17

Brown rice, cooked	1 cup	12
Sunflower seeds	25g	12
Pinto beans, cooked	1 cup	10
Haricot beans, cooked	1 cup	7
Cashew nuts, raw	25g	7
Wholemeal bread	1 slice	3

(Data from the UK Composition of Foods Dataset, https://www.gov.uk/ government/publications/composition-of-foods-integrated-dataset-cofid, and SACN position statement on Selenium and health, https://assets.publishing. service.gov.uk/government/uploads/system/uploads/attachment_data/ file/339431/SACN_Selenium_and_Health_2013.pdf)

This table gives an indication of the selenium content of a selection of plant-based foods in the UK, but it's important to remember that the actual content can vary massively. In fact, the selenium content of foods can vary by up to 100-fold. That's because, much like iodine, the selenium content of crops depends on how much selenium is in the soil, as well as the acidity of the soil. So selenium in food can vary between countries and even between regions within countries. Because in the UK most foods are sourced by retailers from a variety of national and international locations, it makes estimating levels of dietary intake accurately extremely difficult.

You may have also noticed that Brazil nuts are at the top of the table, as an extremely rich source of selenium. In fact they're the richest of any food source, vegan or not. As with all foods, the selenium content can vary greatly depending on the soil conditions in which the Brazil nut tree is grown. For instance, studies show the selenium content in just one Brazil nut (approx. 5g) can vary between 8μg from nuts grown in Bolivia,[80] to 220μg in the Eastern Amazon region.[81] Even within Brazil they can vary by 26-fold.[82] Still, even accounting for this big variation, studies show that consumption of two Brazil nuts a day can improve selenium status as effectively as supplements.[83] But you can see that it would be very easy to exceed the 450μg a day safe upper limit with more than a few Brazil nuts, so be careful not to overdo it.

Although studies show that supplementing with selenium doesn't have direct benefits for aerobic or anaerobic exercise, ensuring enough selenium in the diet is still important to prevent deficiency among athletes with high-intensity and high-volume training. Because of its roles related to antioxidant defences, thyroid hormone production, testosterone metabolism, anti-carcinogenic properties and muscle performance, it's clear that athletes and non-athletes alike need to make sure they're getting enough.

Hopefully, having gone through this chapter, you'll realize just how simple it is to ensure adequate intakes of the key nutrients for vegans and plant-based athletes. In fact, if your diet is already balanced, and based mostly around whole plant foods, you're very likely to already be exceeding the recommended intakes for many of them. But hopefully you now also feel informed about good sources of these key nutrients, and can bear these tips in mind when planning your meals.

You'll probably also have noticed that these nutrients are important for everyone, not just vegans, and that ensuring an adequate intake of them will help promote good health as well as provide your body with what it needs to perform at its best in sports and exercise. In the following chapters we'll go one step further, and look at strategies that can specifically promote faster, more efficient recovery, and provide more energy, power and endurance during performance too.

Then, in Chapter 9, we'll go through creating a balanced meal plan, and you'll see that by including foods from each of the major food groups, it couldn't be simpler to cover most of these key nutrients naturally through the diet. You'll soon become accustomed to the simple guidance, and optimizing your nutrition will become almost automatic as you progress in your sport or activity.

Now we have the fundamentals of how to ensure your plant-based diet is as healthy as it can be, we'll go into more depth in the following chapters on how to adapt your diet to promote optimal strength, fitness, performance and recovery.

CHAPTER 6

RECOVERY

We've seen how effective a plant-based diet can be when it comes to longer-term health benefits and reducing risk for the most prevalent diseases in modern society. Of course, as an athlete, staying healthy is a clear benefit if it means less time out of training due to illness. But nutrition also plays a more specific role in optimizing the beneficial effects of exercise – whether you're a bodybuilder, an endurance athlete, or a recreationally active person looking to improve physical and mental health. Over the following two chapters we'll look at how making the right decisions regarding your plant-based nutrition can result in quicker recovery, maximal muscle growth, and improved performance in a variety of disciplines.

Now you're well versed at weighing up the evidence yourself, you may notice as we go through these chapters that the science behind nutrition for exercise and performance is a little different to the evidence of the longer-term health benefits of a plant-based diet. This is for two main reasons:

1. Fewer participants: Sports nutrition in general tends to be much more specific, and trials are usually conducted on fewer participants than large-scale

population-based studies like many of the ones we've seen so far.

2. Shorter-term: Sports nutrition studies often focus on exercise tasks conducted in laboratory or other closely monitored conditions, meaning that trials are often better controlled, but tend to be relatively short-term. Looking at the effects of dietary patterns over the course of a whole sporting season or even an entire career is much more difficult to control for things like motivation and lifestyle.

Still, there are many good-quality studies showing the numerous performance and recovery benefits of a plant-based diet. I can only imagine this evidence base will continue to expand, because of the rapidly growing interest in the benefits of plant-based diets for exercise performance. We've touched briefly on some of these benefits in Chapter 3, but the following chapters will explore the area in much more detail, incorporate some of the considerations of vegan sports nutrition, and provide some evidence-based practical tips and advice.

HOW AND WHY A VEGAN DIET CAN HELP IMPROVE RECOVERY

As we know, balanced plant-based diets are abundant in vitamins and antioxidants, and these beneficial compounds protect our health, reducing the risk of numerous diseases like cancer and heart disease. But they have another benefit: because they're able to help our bodies neutralize free radicals, they can aid with exercise recovery too. And please don't underestimate the power of recovery, as that's the time where the body enters a state of repair, adaptation and growth. In fact, it could be argued that optimizing our recovery from exercise is just as important as the exercise itself when it comes to improving strength and fitness.

Before we look at the mechanisms behind this element of the diet, and at tips on how to enhance the effect further, we should take a moment to understand the process of exercise-induced free radical production. You'll remember from Chapter 3 that your body is always producing free radicals, especially through processes that involve an oxidation reaction, such as those required for energy production. We need a certain level of free radicals for our health, but an imbalance can lead to damage to our DNA and other important molecules. During exercise, there's a huge increase in free radical production because of the high demand for oxygen required for energy production, particularly within our muscle cells.[1] This notion is, in itself, a paradox – how come exercise, which we all know is a powerful health-promoting act, leads to increases in free radical production that can damage our DNA?

Well, the answer lies in what happens during recovery. First, that increase in free radical production during exercise is relatively short-lived. For instance, a team of researchers measured the exercise-induced DNA damage of ultramarathon runners before, during and after a 50km race that took an average of 7.5 hours to complete. As expected, DNA damage significantly increased mid-race. But, as you can see from the graph on page 114, it returned to the baseline levels by just two hours post-race.[2] Second, oxidative damage decreases during recovery. For instance, in that same study, not only did the level of DNA damage quickly diminish, but it ended up significantly lower than where it started, even six days after the race!

There have been numerous other trials that demonstrate

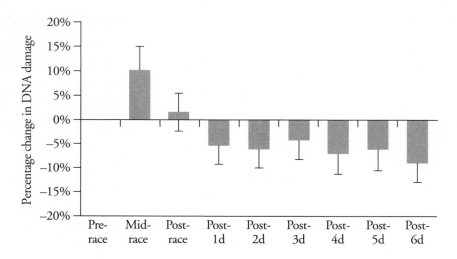

Source: Mastaloudis et al (2004)[3]

this effect, and a recent meta-analysis pooled the results from 19 of them to show that exercise, regardless of the type, intensity, or volume, led to decreased measures of pro-oxidant (DNA-damaging) processes, and that antioxidant indicators increased over time.[4] It seems that the short-lived increase in free radical production when we exercise signals to our bodies to increase the production of our own in-built antioxidant repair systems, so we can better deal with future bouts of exercise[5] (but bear in mind that overtraining, or insufficient rest, can increase oxidative stress to an extent that can outstrip our antioxidant defences, resulting in chronic oxidative stress and subsequent DNA damage. So, always make sure you rest sufficiently between training sessions).

So the short-term oxidative stress induced by exercise is, paradoxically, instrumental in achieving the health benefits from regular exercise. Would an antioxidant-rich diet, then, by reducing exercise-induced oxidative stress, block this adaptation process? Well, in supplement form, yes: researchers put healthy young men on a four-week exercise programme, giving one group vitamins C and E, both potent antioxidants, while the control group received no supplementation. Yes, the supplement group saw lower levels of oxidative damage *during* the exercise, but only the control group saw a boost in their in-built antioxidant defence mechanisms afterwards.[6] Another study looking at antioxidant supplements showed significantly more oxidative stress, and resulting muscle damage, after resistance exercise.[7] It looks like we might need that short-lived stress to stimulate our bodies to adapt.

How about plant-based foods, as opposed to supplements? Do they also blunt this in-built antioxidant adaptation to exercise? Well, it's relatively early days in the research, and studies to date tend to focus on specific foods rather than whole dietary patterns. But current evidence shows us that no, they don't.[8, 9] In fact, it looks like fruit and vegetables provide double benefits: they can help reduce oxidative stress during the exercise, *and* actually enhance the adaptation process, by also ramping up the body's own antioxidant defences. To date, this effect has been shown with antioxidant-rich plant foods like grapes, blueberries, blackcurrants, lemon verbena, watercress and spinach.[10–14] It seems to be the natural phytochemical compounds such as phenolic acids, flavonoids, stilbenes, resveratrol and lignans identified in whole plant foods that have potent antioxidant properties. But, unlike antioxidant supplements, these phytochemicals within whole plant foods can augment the body's in-built adaptive mechanisms.[15]

Levels of oxidative stress seem to have a potent role in the adaptation process following exercise.[16] Reducing oxidative stress with a diet rich in antioxidants can minimize the symptoms of exercise-induced muscle damage, such as muscle pain, soreness, inflammation and reduced muscle function.[17] And improving your recovery is one of the holy grails in sports and exercise nutrition: it means subsequent athletic performance or training quality, particularly when there's limited time to recover between training sessions or competitions, can be optimized. Taken over the course of an entire sporting season or even an entire career, the cumulative benefits can make a big difference to performance.

This effect always reminds me of a distance runner I worked with several years ago. He was in his late 40s and his marathon time had reached a plateau. He put this down to his age, as he'd noticed he couldn't train as often as he used to without constantly feeling sore and stiff. Soon after working with him to devise a plant-based nutrition plan, he reported being able to happily squeeze in an extra run each week without feeling achy, as he had before. The cumulative effect of this extra training resulted in achieving a personal best in a marathon at the end of the season. We're still in touch, and he's since set a new personal best each year over the following three years!

The evidence shows that antioxidants from whole plant foods, but not supplements, can both reduce the oxidative stress during exercise, *and* augment the body's in-built adaptation process by stimulating the production of antioxidant enzymes – thus improving recovery. Meanwhile, increased consumption of red meat, poultry and dairy seems to promote oxidative stress due to the higher levels of saturated fat, animal-based proteins, and haem iron.[18–20] So a plant-based diet can provide double benefits: fewer pro-oxidative animal-based foods, and more antioxidant plant compounds. The evidence so far comes mostly from studies incorporating single plant foods — so imagine the power of an entire diet based around whole plant foods!

Optimizing our antioxidant intake

There's a wide variety of phytochemical compounds with antioxidant properties in varying proportions in all plant foods. The effect of both reducing the risk for many diseases, and reaping the recovery benefits, is not only down to the effect of the individual antioxidants, but also may be the result of antioxidant compounds not yet known, and the synergy of many different antioxidants present in fruits and vegetables working together.[21] So it seems getting the widest variety of antioxidants naturally through our food each day provides us with the greatest rewards. A good way to do this would be to incorporate several colours every day, because some of the most important antioxidant compounds are known to be pigmented and have a characteristic colour. For example, anthocyanins are responsible for red, blue and purple colour in fruits and vegetables. Carotenoids are associated with red or orange colour, and chlorophyll gives the green colour to many vegetables.[22] Including different coloured plants will then naturally promote uptake of the other hundreds of known and unknown antioxidants.

You could try complementing your antioxidant intake with various herbs, spices, teas, and even coffee too. For example, turmeric contains the powerful antioxidant curcumin (absorption of which is increased by up to 2,000% if consumed with black pepper, thanks to its piperine content).[23] Allspice, cinnamon, cloves, saffron, mint, oregano, thyme and sage are all particularly high in antioxidants too. Tea (black and green) and coffee also contribute to antioxidant intake, but bear in mind the advice in Chapter 5 about how they can affect the absorption of some minerals, such as iron.

Let's talk about protein

Protein is an essential component for recovery. It's also vital for sustaining life. Protein is made up of amino acids, which act as the building blocks needed to form the structural basis of most of the body's cells and tissues, such as skeletal muscle, ligaments, bones, skin, hormones, enzymes, and cells in our blood like red blood cells and immune cells (see diagram opposite). But, as you'll see, for the vast majority of people it's incredibly easy to get more than enough protein from plants, without even making a conscious effort. In fact, it's difficult **not** to get enough protein, as long as you're eating enough calories and a varied, balanced, plant-based diet.

We'll discuss optimizing protein intake for optimal recovery later in this chapter, but for now I want to cover how easy it is to meet the requirements for the general population, including recreationally active adults – more for reassurance than anything else. That's because, as any vegan will testify, it's often the first thing people will ask you about your diet: 'But where do you get your protein from?' There seems to be a protein obsession at the moment, driven in part by lucrative weight-loss schemes and promises of easy muscle-building success. But as we'll see, this simply isn't justified.

118

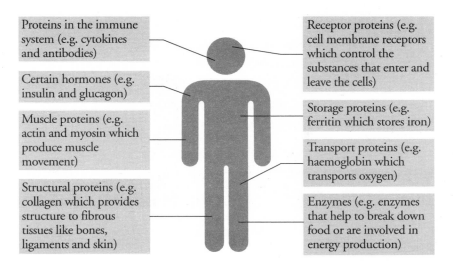

Proteins in the immune system (e.g. cytokines and antibodies)

Certain hormones (e.g. insulin and glucagon)

Muscle proteins (e.g. actin and myosin which produce muscle movement)

Structural proteins (e.g. collagen which provides structure to fibrous tissues like bones, ligaments and skin)

Receptor proteins (e.g. cell membrane receptors which control the substances that enter and leave the cells)

Storage proteins (e.g. ferritin which stores iron)

Transport proteins (e.g. haemoglobin which transports oxygen)

Enzymes (e.g. enzymes that help to break down food or are involved in energy production)

UK Daily Reference Intake: 0.75g protein per kg body-weight daily.

For example, for someone weighing 80kg:

0.75(g) x 80(kg) = 60g protein per day

Or for someone weighing 60kg:

0.75(g) x 60(kg) = 45g protein per day

This is the average requirement, calculated to meet the needs of most (97.5%) of the UK population, and is very easy to achieve on a vegan diet. If you're a recreationally active person who exercises a few times a week, your needs are very likely to be met by this reference intake as long as you're eating enough calories and your diet is varied. Requirements may be lower (than 0.75g/kg) for overweight/ less active people or higher in underweight/more active people. Remember, we'll discuss a little later how you may benefit from increasing your protein intake during more intense training schedules for improving strength and fitness, but for now let's look at a selection of vegan sources of protein to see how easy it is to meet these targets when eating a balanced, varied diet.

FOOD	SERVING SIZE	TYPICAL PROTEIN (g)
Tempeh	120g	23
Lentils, cooked	1 cup	18
Tofu, firm	120g	17
Black beans, cooked	1 cup	15
Chickpeas, cooked	1 cup	15
Chickpea pasta, cooked	1 cup	15
Oats, uncooked	1 cup	10
Peas, cooked	1 cup	9
Wholemeal pasta, cooked	1 cup	8
Quinoa, cooked	1 cup	8
Soya milk	1 cup	7
Spinach, cooked	1 cup	5
Wholemeal bread	1 slice	5
Soya yoghurt	100g	4
Broccoli, cooked	1 cup	4
Nuts, raw	28g	4–7

(Data from USDA FoodData Central https://fdc.nal.usda.gov and individual brand nutrition information.)

Let's look at how simply following general healthy eating guidelines, such as the UK Eatwell Guide,[24] for a day would provide ample amounts of protein:

- **Base meals on higher-fibre starchy foods like potatoes, oats, bread, rice and pasta** – i.e. three portions: approx. **10–20g of protein.**

- **Include some higher-protein foods** – let's say 2 cups of beans, lentils, chickpeas, tofu or tempeh, etc.: approx. **30–40g of protein.**

- **Eat at least 5 portions of fruit and vegetables** (protein varies greatly between different varieties, but let's say a conservative average of 3g per portion): **15g of protein.**

- **Include some dairy alternatives** (soya options contain much more protein than other dairy alternatives, so let's say just one serving is soya-based): approx. **5g of protein.**

Daily total = 60–80g of protein.

You can see how simply eating a balanced diet, even without making a conscious effort, can provide ample amounts of protein for most people. And remember, if you're more active, you're likely to fuel your training by eating more foods like starchy grains, fruits and vegetables, which would contribute to an even higher protein intake without even trying. We'll delve much deeper into this shortly, but for now it's important to know that for most people, simply eating a balanced vegan diet will provide more than enough protein.

Amino acid profile

Proteins are made up of 20 amino acids, 9 of which are 'essential' because our bodies can't produce them on their own, so they need to be provided by the foods we eat. Some amino acids are classified as 'conditionally essential' as they can be made by the body, but are considered essential in times of growth because the body can't make them at a rate necessary to support growth, so they need to be provided by the foods we eat during these times.

Animal foods (meat, poultry, fish, eggs and dairy) and some plant foods (quinoa and soy) contain all the amino acids, but most plant foods are low in at least one amino acid. However, a varied and balanced vegan diet consisting of a variety of whole plant foods will contain all the amino acids necessary. For example, legumes tend to be high in the amino acid lysine, but are low in methionine, whereas most grains are high in methionine and low in lysine. So a meal of beans on toast (legume with grain) will provide the full range of amino acids. In the context of an overall diet consisting of pulses, legumes, whole grains, nuts, seeds, fruit and vegetables, you can rest assured you'll be getting plenty of each individual amino acid.

As well as this, your body can draw from its 'free amino acid pool' which comes from food consumed in the previous meal, and because there's a constant turnover of cells, and therefore protein, in the body. See the diagram opposite, which shows how exogenous (dietary) and endogenous (body) proteins contribute to the free amino acid pool. The rate of cell turnover in various tissues, contributing to the endogenous sources of amino acids, are shown in the table on page 124. So, if for any reason a certain meal you eat is low in a particular amino acid, your body can draw from this 'pool' to balance things out. That's why the old misconception that vegans needed to eat specific combinations of plant proteins within each meal was dispelled many years ago[25] and has been replaced by advice to simply consume a variety of plant-based protein sources throughout the day.[26]

What's more, most meals do tend to naturally combine plant protein sources anyway. For example, you're unlikely to just have a bowl of rice on its own – you'd be more likely to eat it with some beans or other legumes and vegetables. So although you don't have to worry about combining plant proteins at each meal, most meals nonetheless

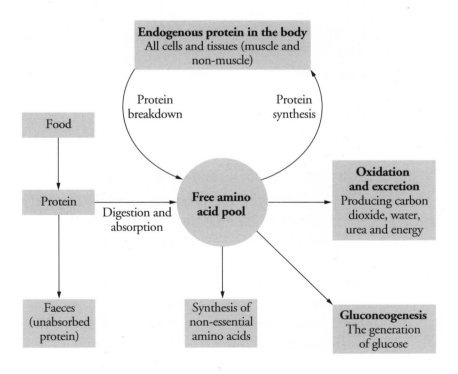

Cell type	Estimated cell turnover rate
Bone marrow	3 days
Colon	3–4 days
Spleen	8 days
Oesophagus	10 days
Endometrium	13 days
Urinary bladder	49 days
Salivary gland	60 days
Skin epidermis	64 days
Lung	200 days
Kidney	270 days
Liver	327 days
Adipose tissue	2,448 days
Skeletal muscle	5,510 days
Heart muscle	25,300 days
Brain neurons	32,850 days

Source: Seim, Ma & Gladyshev (2016)[27]

naturally provide complementary mixtures of the essential amino acids.

So hopefully the message regarding protein is clear – for most people, eating a healthy, balanced vegan diet with plenty of variation will provide ample amounts of protein. In fact, surveys of vegan populations from Europe and America show that protein intakes average between 62g and 82g a day, well above the 50g a day which is often taken as a very approximate daily reference value (for example on food packaging).[28–32] By following the healthy balanced dietary recommendations throughout this book, you too will be taking in plenty of protein.

Ways to maximize muscle protein synthesis

Skeletal muscles (the muscles that move our skeleton, rather than smooth muscle in the walls of internal organs, for instance) have astonishing levels of plasticity in how they can adapt to cope with the demands of exercise. It's not just a case of muscles growing when demand increases, but even the type of exercise dictates what specific adaptations the muscle cells make. For instance, endurance training results mainly in increases in the number and size of the mitochondria, which generate most of the energy within our cells, while strength training promotes muscle growth and strength through increases in muscle fibre volume.[33] So muscle protein synthesis and promoting other muscular adaptations isn't something just bodybuilders should be interested in; it's important for all athletes, ranging from ultramarathon runners to powerlifters, and everyone in between.

To recognize what we can do to influence the growth and adaptation of our muscles, it's important to understand some basic principles in muscle metabolism. Principally, there are two processes that simultaneously occur to keep all skeletal muscle in a constant state of turnover:

- Muscle protein synthesis (MPS) – the creation of new muscle proteins, i.e. building muscle.

- Muscle protein breakdown (MPB) – the degradation of muscle proteins into their constituent amino acids, i.e. breaking down muscle tissue.

This turnover process is crucial for the constant repair and remodelling of muscle proteins, especially important following exercise when there is damage to some of the muscle proteins and we want to promote repair and growth. In healthy active people, this skeletal muscle turnover exists in a state of dynamic equilibrium: when in a fasted state, breakdown

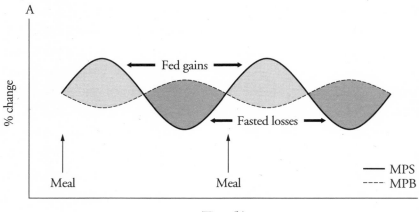

Time (h)

exceeds synthesis, but when in a fed state, synthesis exceeds breakdown. So, over the course of a normal day, muscle turnover is in a state of balance – see the graph above.

In response to exercise, MPS is transiently increased, while MPB may increase slightly, or remain the same, depending on the exercise and other nutrition factors (we'll discuss the role of nutrition on MPB shortly). The result is, on a cumulative basis, that those increases in MPS after regular bouts of exercise 'drive' adaptation to training and overall increases in muscle mass (see the graph opposite).

This elevated MPS response to resistance training can last up to around 48 hours in untrained adults,[34] while athletes who are more acclimatized to training might expect MPS to return to baseline levels after around 36 hours.[35] It's not within the remit of this book to discuss the numerous

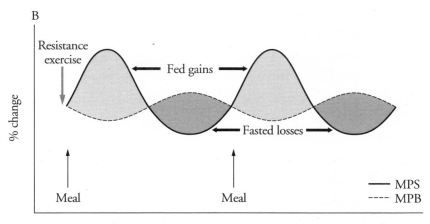

exercise variables that can affect MPS (such as number of sets, reps, rest periods and training frequency) other than to say it very much depends on what your goals are or which sport you're training for. We will, however, look at the nutritional considerations to help optimize MPS and (to a lesser extent) minimize MPB.

The main way to maximize exercise-induced MPS is by increasing protein intake, and ensuring a sufficient caloric intake. However, as you'll see, the amount of protein we need to see this effect might be lower than you think, and it's easy to achieve this level on a vegan diet.

We discussed protein requirements for the general population earlier in the chapter. Remember, this level, of 0.75g/kg/day, has been calculated to meet the needs of 97.5% of the population. If you're a recreationally active person, perhaps exercising moderately 2–3 times a week, this is likely to be plenty for you. A classic study from the early 1990s illustrates this point perfectly: researchers took two groups of males – strength training athletes (training 5 or more days a week), and more sedentary subjects. They randomly assigned both of these groups to one of three diets: one provided the Canadian reference intake for protein (which is a little higher than in the UK at 0.86g/kg/day), one provided 1.4g/kg/day, and the other provided 2.4g/kg/day. The researchers found that the diet providing 1.4g/kg/day did increase whole-body protein synthesis – but only in the strength training athletes.[36] In other words, unless you're training regularly, increasing your protein intake above normal levels won't make any difference to how much muscle you synthesize.

Interestingly, the study showed that even in the strength training athletes, increasing the protein intake to 2.4g/kg/day made no further difference compared to 1.4g/kg/day – so it appears there's a limit to how much protein is beneficial for increasing exercise-induced MPS.

A recent meta-analysis confirmed this theory. Researchers took data from 49 studies assessing protein intake, and found that during periods of resistance exercise training, increasing protein intake does indeed significantly enhance changes in muscle strength and size. However, this effect plateaus as protein intake increases, and they found that levels above ~1.6g/kg/day made no further difference to muscle growth.[37] Anything above this, it appears, would be a waste of time and (seeing as higher protein foods are often more expensive) money. In fact, depending on your goals, it could even be detrimental, as excess protein in the diet either gets used for energy or stored as fat.

The optimal level of protein also depends on your training type. Some recommendations suggest endurance athletes aim for around 1.2g/kg/day, while athletes emphasizing strength and power, such as bodybuilders and powerlifters, might require as much as 2.0g/kg/day, according to the American College of Sports Medicine and the Academy of Nutrition and Dietetics.[38] Most individual and team sports require a combination of aerobic with short bursts of power, and so a range between these two levels would likely be suitable. Requirements are likely to be lower for people who are overweight or obese, and there's evidence that well-trained, experienced athletes require less than people first initiating an exercise programme. Requirements can even vary for individual athletes, depending on periodized training schedules and specific training sessions. However, the ranges advised for athletes can still be used as an approximate guide. You can estimate your overall average daily protein requirements using the table below:

Your body weight in kg (lb divided by 2.2)	___ (a)
Estimated protein requirement - 0.75 (recreationally active) - 1.2 (endurance-focused athlete) - 1.6 (strength-focused athlete) - 2.0 (upper range for strength training athlete)	___ (b1) to ___ (b2)
Overall range (a x b1 and a x b2)	___ to ___

Let's give an example of a well-trained rugby fly half, weighing 80kg. Training is likely to be a combination of endurance and strength training, so a range of 1.2–1.6g/kg/day would likely be suitable:

80 x 1.2 = 96g of protein per day (suitable when training emphasizes endurance and skill-based exercise).

80 x 1.6 = 128g of protein per day (more appropriate following gym-based strength training).

129

It should be noted that the timing of protein intake is also of importance. It's a commonly held belief that consuming protein immediately after training is most effective for promoting muscle growth, but two recent meta-analyses of randomized controlled trials show that consuming protein around training sessions makes no significant difference.[39, 40] What both meta-analyses do show, however, is that total protein intake is the most important factor. Does this mean we shouldn't have a high-protein meal, or a vegan protein shake, straight after training? Not necessarily – they can still be helpful for the following reasons:

- It's a simple method to help contribute to your total daily protein intake, the most important factor for increasing MPS.
- It's easy to do, and can be a rewarding way to end a hard training session.
- Even though the meta-analyses mentioned show that on average it doesn't make a difference, everyone is different and it might still theoretically have a small positive effect, so you won't feel like you're missing out.
- A post-exercise snack or meal often also contains some carbohydrates which (as we'll discuss shortly) can limit MPB.

Another note on protein timing is that spreading your protein intake throughout the course of the day appears to be much more effective for promoting MPS than fewer, bigger meals. Studies show that consuming 20–30g of protein (suitable for the typical range of athlete body sizes) in several meals or snacks distributed throughout the day will promote MPS more effectively than concentrating protein intake into one or two larger meals.[41, 42] High doses (i.e. 40g of protein or more) have not yet been shown to further enhance MPS, and may only be suitable for the largest of athletes.[43] So, if your aim is to promote muscle strength and growth, a beneficial diet pattern would be to incorporate high-protein vegan foods into your breakfast, lunch, dinner and snacks throughout the day. If you refer back to the graph on page 127, you can see how this will enhance MPS optimally through the fed periods over the 36–48 hours after training.

Seeing as your overnight sleep is the longest period you won't eat, it also makes sense to consume some protein before bed. This will promote one last increase in MPS before your long overnight fasting period during sleep. This strategy has been shown to be effective for both acute post-exercise recovery[44] and long-term improvements in muscle mass and strength gains during strength training programmes.[45] A large meal just before bed may impair your sleep, so a high-protein smaller evening snack instead could be beneficial.

I also want to mention a topic of debate regarding plant-based protein: its digestibility. The theory is that the rate of digestion and absorption of protein from plant foods can be lower than animal-based proteins, because plant foods more often contain nutrients that can reduce the digestibility of protein by, for example, inhibiting certain enzymes in the gut that break down proteins so that they can be absorbed. Much of the evidence adding to this concern is based on historical studies on rats, or in humans using dated, less accurate methods.[46] More recent studies show that the difference is much less than previously thought, if any. For example, more precise methods of assessment showed the digestibility of soy protein isolate, pea protein flour, cooked rice and wheat flour to be 89–92%, similar to those found for eggs (91%) and meat (90–94%).[47] And a meta-analysis of nitrogen balance studies in humans (a method to study protein metabolism) showed no difference between three separate groups: protein from animal, vegetable or mixed sources.[48]

Still, the evidence on the difference in digestibility between plant and animal protein sources is far from concrete, and varies depending on research technique, and from person to person depending on lifestyle factors and dietary patterns. Although probably not necessary, a prudent approach could be to aim for around a 10% higher protein intake to account for this.

The focus of this section so far has been on promoting MPS, because we know that exercise and nutrition can influence MPS to a much greater degree than it can for MPB. Nevertheless, minimizing exercise-induced MPB could still contribute a little to the overall gains in muscle strength and size. The key nutritional factor to minimize MPB is insulin, which, as you may remember from Chapter 3, is released by pancreatic cells in response to raised blood sugar levels. In fact, a recent meta-analysis showed that while insulin doesn't affect MPS, it does significantly reduce MPB, resulting in an increased net balance of muscle protein acquisition.[49] However, relatively low levels of insulin are needed to have this effect,[50] so a typical high-protein plant-based meal or even a vegan protein shake is likely to induce enough of an insulin rise to significantly reduce MPB. This could be another reason why eating a mixed meal shortly after training may have some benefits. In any case, some MPB is important for muscle cell remodelling and growth following exercise,[51] so we wouldn't want to prevent it altogether anyway.

Considering protein supplements

It's relatively easy for most vegan athletes to meet their protein requirements using whole plant foods, especially when you consider that athletes tend to naturally have a much higher overall food intake in order to meet their increased energy demands anyway. If you're concerned that you may not be reaching the levels necessary to optimize MPS, you could try tracking your protein intake over a couple of days using a free web-based nutrition tracking app such as Cronometer – you might be pleasantly surprised at how the protein in bread, pasta, grains and vegetables, on top of the high-protein foods like legumes and tofu, all quickly adds up. If you find your intake is below your estimated requirements, simply try adding 1–3 portions of the high-protein plant foods listed on page 120 to your meals and snacks. Chapter 10 is also filled with protein-packed meal ideas if you're in need of inspiration for high-protein recipes.

Another option for convenience is protein supplements, usually in the form of nutritional shakes or bars. Historically, the taste of vegan protein shakes left much to be desired, but in recent years some very palatable, even tasty brands have emerged. The best options are those made from a blend of protein sources, such as pea, hemp, and rice proteins – this ensures a full range of the amino acids. But you'd be much better off to first ensure a balanced daily diet (such as at least three meals daily comprised of a variety of foods from each of the major food groups, consuming enough energy to support your level of physical activity, and keeping properly hydrated), as these dietary fundamentals are far more important for your growth than protein supplements. Shakes and bars should never be used to replace a varied and balanced diet, but can come in handy to augment the diet for some athletes with particularly high requirements.

It should also be mentioned that using a plant-based protein shake is no reflection on the ability to get enough protein on a vegan diet, and is simply a matter of convenience – the same reason it's very typical to see meat-eaters drinking whey protein shakes after a gym session!

We've reviewed how the high antioxidative qualities of a plant-based diet can help with recovery, and ways we can tweak our diet to further enhance this effect. Hopefully you now also feel reassured about the big protein question, and can take away some useful tips to enhance muscle protein synthesis. These aspects of recovery are vital to seeing long-term improvements in both strength- and endurance-orientated sports. Faster recovery is also crucial if you're training hard frequently, or competing in a sport where there's limited rest between stages or competitions, such as multi-stage cycle events.

But what about improving performance in the more immediate sense: can a plant-based diet give you the edge here too? And are there ways we can optimize our diet to get the most out of key training sessions or during competitions? The answer to both of these questions is yes, and we'll delve right into the reasons in the next chapter.

CHAPTER 7

PERFORMANCE

HOW AND WHY A VEGAN DIET
CAN HELP IMPROVE PERFORMANCE

Hopefully now you can fully appreciate the importance of recovery when it comes to sports performance, as that's the time when the body is adapting, repairing and growing. But what about physical performance *during* the exercise – can that be affected by eating a plant-based diet too?

One approach to answer this question could be to discuss the large (and fast-growing) number of vegan athletes and sportspeople who are surpassing their competitors. Just a small selection of athletes who have adopted a plant-based diet, and a summary of their achievements, is listed in the table below.

ATHLETE	DISCIPLINE	ACHIEVEMENTS SINCE ADOPTING PLANT-BASED DIET
Emil Voigt	Athletics	Gold medal in the 5-mile race at the 1908 London Olympics
Murray Rose	Swimming	Four Olympic gold medals for swimming in 1956 and 1960, setting new world records for the 400, 800, and 1500-metre freestyle

Carl Lewis	Athletics	Won the 100-metre sprint at the 1991 World Championships, setting a new world record
Fiona Oakes	Distance running	Won the Antarctic Ice Marathon and the North Pole Marathons in 2013, and set four world records for marathon running
Serena Williams	Tennis	Won her 23rd Grand Slam singles title in 2017, the most won by any player in modern tennis
Lewis Hamilton	Formula 1	Won his sixth World Title in 2019, world record holder for all-time career points and most points in a season (2019)
Kyrie Irving	Basketball	The first player in NBA history to score 50 points in a team debut for the Brooklyn Nets in 2019
Novak Djokovic	Tennis	Won his 17th Grand Slam title in 2020, ranked ATP world number one in men's singles tennis in 2020
Tyrann Mathieu	American football	Won the 2020 Superbowl with the Kansas City Chiefs

Citing the achievements of these plant-based athletes is of course not a scientific approach – it's anecdotal by its very nature. It is, however, fascinating, and certainly shows that a plant-based diet doesn't hold you back, and can provide the nutrition you need to support achieving world-class performance in a range of disciplines.

The first scientific studies assessing the effectiveness of plant-based diets for performance were conducted in the early 1900s. Some of these studies directly compared plant-based athletes with omnivorous athletes (matched for age, size and weight, etc.), and found that the plant-based athletes had considerably more strength endurance in exercises such as leg raises, horizontal arm holds, and grip strength.[1, 2] Several more recent studies comparing the performance of plant-based with omnivorous athletes have also found better results in those following a plant-based diet, particularly when it comes to cardio-respiratory fitness.[3] The problem with these studies, though, is that they aren't at all robust in their design – in particular, there's no random assignment of participants to the plant-based or meat-eating groups. A possible explanation for the superior physical capacity of the plant-based partici-pants could be an increased sense of drive and grit, due to the added motivation to out-perform their meat-eating rivals. This is a phenomenon I've experienced personally, and many of my clients have reported having similar motivations. I'm sure many of you reading this will relate to this too! A prime example is the record-breaking distance runner Fiona Oakes, who was quoted as not particularly enjoying running, but her love for animals motivated her to train harder than her competitors so she could win races, set records, and use her platform to promote the power of plant-based diets.

The alternative to recruiting long-term vegans, who may have that extra determination to train harder, or do well in the tests, would be to take omnivorous participants and randomly assign them to either continue their meat-eating diet, or pro-vide them with a plant-based diet that's matched for calories and macronutrients. Studies taking this approach have found that although a vegan diet doesn't have any adverse effects on performance, it provides no benefits either. A systematic review combined results from seven such randomized controlled trials and showed that this was the case for muscular power, muscu-lar strength and aerobic performance.[4] However, a serious flaw with this approach is that it's difficult to conduct this kind of experiment for a long time – studies prescribing participants to a specific diet for extended periods would be expensive and run the risk of lower compliance to the diet. So, research of this nature tends to be short-term. For instance, the studies included in the systematic review mentioned above varied in length of between just four days and twelve weeks.

On top of this, these short-term controlled trials tend to simply focus on the completion of an exercise task under controlled conditions in a laboratory, which can differ greatly from real sporting scenarios, such as a player's energy, speed, and skill during a real-life football match. Any athlete will testify that peak performance in sport depends on countless factors and often takes years of training, eating, and resting optimally to achieve.

So you can see that devising a robust study to prove the benefits of plant-based diets to athletic performance is very difficult to do. While both existing methods have their flaws, until researchers are able to design a study that can somehow make comparisons more accurately, those studies showing improved performance in long-standing vegans when compared to matched omnivores should certainly be considered in the equation.

We can also consider the wealth of mechanistic evidence that shows why plant-based athletes can have the upper hand – looking at the possible biological processes which could result in improved performance. For example, as mentioned in the last chapter, the high levels of antioxidants in fruits, vegetables, pulses and grains help reduce exercise-induced oxidative stress. However, as well as promoting recovery after exercise, they've been shown to also delay the onset of muscle fatigue during the exercise itself.[5]

A plant-based diet also tends to be much richer in dietary flavanols – a class of phytochemicals with antioxidant properties found in many different fruits and vegetables. These have been shown in various studies to improve maximal oxygen uptake (VO2 max), enhance fat oxidation, reduce the oxygen cost of exercise, and help the muscles use ATP, the energy currency of our cells, more efficiently.[6-8] Flavanols can also induce improvements in the elasticity of the blood vessels, known as vasodilation, resulting in a reduction in blood pressure during exercise which can decrease the workload of the heart. Collectively, all these effects can also help to improve exercise efficiency, delay the onset of fatigue, and increase the capacity of endurance exercise.[9]

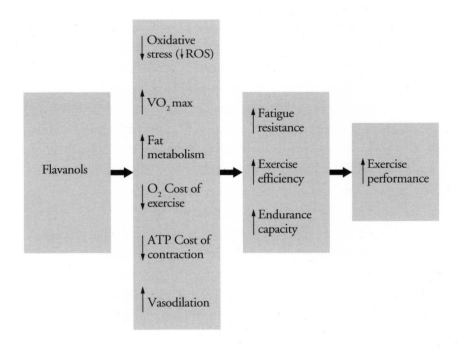

Source: Al-Dashti et al (2018)[10]

A plant-based diet can also improve the fluidity of your blood. If you think of your blood as liquid within a plumbing network, then you can imagine that thinner, more fluid liquid will flow through the piping system much more quickly and efficiently than thicker, viscous liquid would. This improved blood fluidity has been shown both in studies of long-standing vegans/vegetarians, and in more controlled studies, within just 6 weeks of adopting a plant-based diet.[11–14] The mechanisms behind this effect aren't yet known exactly, but are likely to be complex, and at least in part due to the increased antioxidant intake and lower saturated fat intake of plant-based diets.[15] However the biological mechanisms work, the result is blood that can flow through your capillaries more efficiently and transport and deliver oxygen to your muscles more easily during exercise.[16]

Continuing with the plumbing analogy, another effective way of improving the flow of liquid is to enhance the piping system itself. Within the body, this can be achieved by improving vascular function. This refers to the control of blood flow, which is usually regulated by a balance between vasoconstriction (which makes our blood vessels narrow) and vasodilation (which makes our blood vessels relax and widen). During exercise, there's a substantial increase in vasodilator signals formed in the active muscle tissue, which helps to widen the skeletal muscle blood vessels, to increase blood flow and oxygen supply to muscles when they need it most during exercise.[17, 18] Dietary nitrates and nitrites, rich in plant foods, can help to improve this vascular function. How? They provide a source for the production of nitric oxide, which signals to the smooth muscle surrounding blood vessels to relax, thus increasing blood flow. In fact, a systematic review looking at beetroot juice, very rich in nitrates, assessed 23 studies and showed that it increases levels of nitric oxide, and results in improved muscle efficiency, increased time to exhaustion, and improved cardiorespiratory performance at anaerobic intensities.[19]

The foods highest in nitrates and nitrites include celery, cress, chervil, lettuce, beetroot, spinach and rocket.[20] Fennel, leek, parsley, celeriac and Chinese cabbage are also great sources. Processed meats also often contain nitrites, which are added to preserve the meat, enhance its flavour, and impart the 'desirable' pink colour. However, in processed meats, the nitrites react with the amines in the meat during processing, curing, storage and cooking to form nitrosamines, which are known carcinogens.[21] As discussed in Chapter 3, this could be one of the main reasons why processed meat is so strongly linked with colorectal cancer. On the other hand, nutrients contained in fruits and vegetables, such as vitamin C and certain phenolic compounds, inhibit the formation of nitrosamines from the nitrates they contain.[22] So in plant foods, much more of the nitrates are converted to nitric oxide, boosting vascular function in athletes.

One final, slightly simpler performance benefit of a plant-based diet we'll look at here is its tendency to be higher in carbohydrates. Seeing as carbohydrates come almost exclusively from plants, it's easy to get plenty on a vegan diet, with pulses, whole grains, and starchy fruit and vegetables all being great sources.

Carbohydrates provide the main fuel for the brain and central nervous system, and are a key substrate for muscular work, where it can support exercise over a large range of intensities because it can be used by both aerobic and anaerobic pathways.[23] In fact, carbohydrate is the only fuel that can sustain moderate- to high-level effort that's required in most sports or athletic endeavours, and research shows that high-carb diets delay the onset of fatigue[24] and maintain power output during both continuous and intermittent exercise (including variable speed running required in many team sports).[25] Practical examples of this have been shown in studies comparing high vs low carbohydrate diets in athletes: with the high-carb diets, athletes were able to run faster in the final 400m of a 10k race,[26] and footballers covered more distance at all speeds, from jogging to all-out sprinting, during a football game.[27] For anyone who takes part in stop-and-go sports such as football, basketball, rugby, hockey, boxing or tennis, this means you'll be able to train or play for longer before feeling fatigued, and can also maintain your ability to perform explosive movements like tackling, sprinting, jumping, serving and punching towards the end of the game.

Translating theory into practice

We've seen that various aspects of a plant-based diet could provide significant performance benefits when done right. All the theory in this section boils down to very simple advice – we should be aiming to incorporate as wide a variety of whole plant foods as possible in order to see the powerful benefits of their antioxidants, flavanols, nitrates, and carbohydrate content, all while minimizing saturated fat intake (while most saturated fat comes from animal foods, coconut and palm oils are also concentrated sources).

GETTING ENOUGH ENERGY TO FUEL A HIGHLY ACTIVE EXERCISE SCHEDULE

The relatively low-calorie density of most plant foods is a bonus for most people who are looking for a sustainable way to manage their weight. But what about athletes, burning through vast amounts of energy throughout their training and competitions? Can a plant-based diet provide enough calories and energy to fuel their highly active exercise schedule and keep them performing at their best?

Some athletes undergoing very high levels of intense physical training may require well over 5,000 calories a day. This is certainly true for some of the larger athletes I work with, such as professional rugby forwards weighing over 120 kilos, burning vast amounts of energy through hours of vigorous training each day. Similar extreme energy demands may be required by long-distance endurance athletes such as ultra-marathon runners and athletes training for and competing in distance stage bike races such as the Tour de France. This will be more than the needs for most athletes, and we'll talk more about why I don't recommend counting calories in Chapter 9 – but I've mentioned this to highlight just how much energy can be required in some situations. If you're an athlete with particularly high energy demands and find it hard to eat enough to fuel your intense training regimen, then following some of the simple strategies in this section might be helpful, probably essential, to your success in both training and competitions.

A key reason is that getting enough calories, in order to match energy expenditure, ensures that more amino acids are used for muscle protein synthesis, rather than being oxidized and used for energy, through a process called gluconeogenesis.[28, 29] When energy – particularly carbohydrate – intake is low, your body needs to pull resources from elsewhere in order to keep up glycogen levels (the body's preferred energy source for moderate-to-high levels of activity required in most sport and athletic endeavours). Some come from the metabolism of fats, but some will come from amino acids. In other words, not getting enough energy will effectively eat into your muscle and you'd require even higher levels of protein in the diet to compensate for this.[30]

Looking at the more immediate effects of consuming insufficient energy, a caloric deficit can also negatively affect cognition, mood, and self-reported exertion during exercise.[31] So the chances are if you go training with low glycogen stores due to a caloric deficit, your decision-making won't be as agile, the training will feel harder, and you'll likely not cover as much ground. As you can see, making sure you get enough energy is important for both short-term performance and long-term adaptations to your training.

I don't encourage any of my clients to count their calories, whether they're looking to gain muscle mass or lose weight, for many reasons, including the following:

- It's very inaccurate – people tend to significantly misreport their diet.[32] In fact, studies show that even trained dieticians incorrectly report their own caloric intake.[33]

- Caloric needs fluctuate significantly from day to day – factors such as training schedules, daily activities, and quality/quantity of sleep, all make setting a precise daily calorie target an arbitrary exercise.

- It's time-consuming – especially when calculating home-cooked foods (which should make up the majority of your diet), as you have to weigh every ingredient, enter each one into a calorie tracking app, and divide by the number of portions. The time spent doing this could be spent much more productively – training, relaxing, sleeping, or seeing friends and family.

A far more practical way to assess whether you're consuming enough energy is to ask yourself the following questions:

- Do you find it hard to keep weight on?

- Do you lack the energy to get you through your training?

- Do you regularly crave calorie-dense, processed foods high in sugar and fat (chocolate, cake, biscuits, etc.), despite trying to eat healthy foods most of the time?

If you answer yes to one or more of these questions, then the chances are you're not getting enough energy from your diet to match the energy you spend exercising. Here are some simple tips you could try, to up your energy intake:

1. Try replacing some of your whole grains with lower-fibre versions. I know this is counter-intuitive for most people, but if you're burning high amounts of energy through intense training, then a diet focused on whole grains can make it difficult to meet your energy and carbohydrate needs, because of the low energy-density of these foods.
   This is an issue several of my clients have faced in the past: sometimes they'd been burning through

an additional 2,000+ calories a day during their training, and trying to make healthy food choices by always opting for whole wheat pasta, brown rice, and whole grain breads with their meals. The high fibre content of these foods, however, meant their stomachs were quickly getting full before they were able to eat enough to balance their extreme energy output.

The advice in this scenario is to relax on the whole grains – by all means still include them, but try also incorporating some white pasta, white rice, white bread, or peeled potatoes (e.g. mashed or roasted), as your carbohydrate sources, to replace some of the whole grains to help increase the caloric density of meals (incidentally, this approach can also help with people experiencing excessive gas or bloating caused by too much fibre in the diet).

2. You could also try replacing some whole fruit with fruit juices. Again, this advice might come as a surprise for some, as general nutrition guidelines, such as the UK Eatwell Guide, suggest limiting intake of fruit juice and to aim to eat whole fruits instead. That's because most people don't consume enough fibre, and most people need to manage or reduce their weight. But if you struggle to keep weight on, fruit juice can provide a more concentrated source of calories than eating whole fruits, which can be useful for meeting the high energy demands of an intense training programme. Also, if you're eating a plant-based diet, the chances are you're already getting plenty of fibre through

eating lots of pulses, vegetables, some grains, nuts and seeds. A good balance would be to still eat some whole fruit but to help top up caloric intake by incorporating some fruit juice into the diet too if necessary.

3. Include more fats from whole plant foods. Hopefully after reading the section on omega-3 in Chapter 5, you'll be regularly including foods like flaxseeds, hemp seeds, chia seeds, and walnuts in your daily diet, if you weren't already. Other healthy whole food fat sources include avocados, tahini (sesame seed paste), other nuts and seeds, and nut butters such as peanut, cashew and almond. Fats are a concentrated source of energy: one gram of fat contains 9 calories, compared to 4 calories in one gram of carbohydrates or protein. So upping your intake of these healthy fat sources is an easy way to increase the caloric content of your meals. The spicy seed mix (see page 293) or the high-protein oat bars (see page 297) are excellent examples of adding nuts and seeds to provide a calorie-dense, high-protein snack. You could also try adding lightly toasted nuts and seeds, or dressings made from whole plant fat sources (such as those on pages 264–8) to stir-fries, salads, or a simple bowl of veggies, rice and beans. As well as fats, these whole foods provide a huge variety of other important nutrients – numerous vitamins, minerals, phytochemicals, and some protein and fibre. Oils contain fat but are much lower in these other nutrients, which is why I recommend getting the majority of your fats through whole plant foods. Again, a relaxed

approach is best – a little oil can greatly enhance the taste of cooking, especially when sautéing and roasting vegetables. But if you get the majority of your fats through whole plant foods, they'll come packaged with countless other important nutrients and protein.

4. Try your hand at smoothies – it's easy to make them very energy- and nutrient-dense. Page 238 has a great example of a high-calorie smoothie, which includes bananas, oats, nut butter, dates, greens and vegan protein powder to provide a total of over 1,000 calories in one delicious drink. Even without going to quite this extreme, it's easy to make a 500-calorie smoothie by just combining fruit, vegetables, and some seeds or nuts – perfect to have alongside your regular breakfast or for a mid-morning snack to boost your energy intake.

Using these tips can help you easily meet the demands of even the most energy-intensive training regimens on a vegan diet, and has helped clients of mine ranging from professional rugby players to ultra-distance runners to meet their extreme energy demands. It can be tempting to rely heavily on sweets, chocolate and cookies to meet high energy needs, and there should certainly be no hard-and-fast restrictive rules on these kinds of foods (I for one am a big dessert fan). So again, a relaxed approach is best, but focusing primarily on the tips above is a great way to up your energy intake while also providing some important nutrition – vitamins, minerals, protein, antioxidants and phytochemicals, which hopefully you know by now are incredibly important for both long-term health and immediate performance and recovery benefits.

NUTRITION TIMING FOR
SPORTS PERFORMANCE

Now you have some tools in your armoury to help you fuel a highly active training schedule, it's useful to know what to eat around your exercise to perform at your best. Getting the right fuel in before, and sometimes during, your competition or key training sessions is critical for optimizing your performance. In fact, overlooking this can negate all the hard work put in by athletes and sportspeople in their training and efforts to eat well at other times. Optimizing your nutrition timing can delay the onset of fatigue, maintain optimal outputs in terms of strength, power and endurance, while providing your brain with the fuel it needs to keep you focused, alert and motivated throughout your sporting event. This can be especially important towards the end of a race, event, or game when it often matters most. This can all be done using strategies to avoid (or limit/delay) glycogen depletion, dehydration, electrolyte imbalances and gastrointestinal discomfort/upset.

Let's begin with hydration. It might not be the first thing to come to mind when considering your nutrition for sports performance, but I would argue that perhaps it should — partly because it's such a simple aspect to address, but also because hydration status affects mood, reaction times, alertness and performance in both endurance and power activities so significantly.[34–38] Of course, the amount you need to drink will depend on the individual, the type of exercise, and the environment (e.g. heat and humidity). When we exercise, we sweat — because it's our main way of dissipating the extra metabolic heat generated by the working muscles. If we sweat

149

a lot without replacing the fluids by hydrating properly, it can lead to a decrease in our blood volume (known as hypovolae-mia) which can lead to cardiovascular strain, increased glyco-gen use, and altered metabolic and nervous system function. As you can imagine, this can seriously impact performance of both aerobic and explosive activities as well as technical skills. Not to mention increased risk of cramps, headaches and even heatstroke. Here's some simple guidance to help make sure you keep optimally hydrated:

Before: In the 24-hour lead-up to an event or key training session, try to ensure you drink generous amounts of fluid, to keep well hydrated. You can monitor your hydration status using your urine colour – it should be a pale-yellow colour. Then, in the 2–4 hour period before exercise, 5–10ml/kg of fluid can help you hydrate but will allow enough time for urine output to return to normal.[39] So for an athlete weigh-ing 80kg, that equates to 400–800ml fluid (5–10 x 80) in the 2–4 hour window before the event.

During: You ideally want to drink enough to maintain your body weight (nearly all weight lost during most exercise is water). The routine measurement of pre- and post-exercise body weights to determine your own sweat rate can be really useful to determine your own fluid replacement strategy, so you're not guessing during important events. If maintaining your body weight isn't possible because of sporting rules or practicality, you should drink as much as you can to prevent losses of more than 2% of body weight (e.g. no more than 1.6kg loss for an 80kg athlete). This can usually be achieved by drinking small amounts every 15–20 minutes. Drinking cold drinks (0.5°C) can help reduce core temperature and therefore improve performance in the heat, and adding fla-vour to drinks (e.g. fruit squash) can increase palatability and encourage fluid intake. With all this being said, do be careful not to overhydrate, as this can cause serious health problems – you should not gain weight during exercise as this could indicate that you're drinking too much fluid.

After: Most athletes finish training or competitions in a fluid deficit, so the goal is to adequately and safely rehydrate during the recovery period. The American College of Sports Medicine recommends drinking up to 1.5 litres of fluid for every kilo lost during exercise – that's because sweat losses and obligatory urine losses continue in the post-exercise phase, so effective rehydration requires an intake of a greater volume of fluid than the amount lost during exercise.[40]

While on the topic of hydration, electrolyte balance is another important factor for some athletes, as they're critical for maintaining fluid balance and blood pressure control. The main electrolyte we need to watch during exercise is sodium, because we lose substantial amounts through our sweat, but others include potassium, calcium and magnesium. In general, you need to think about electrolyte balance during exercise where large sweat losses occur, for instance:

1. If you're exercising for over 2 hours.
2. If you have a high sweat rate (over 1.2 litres per hour).
3. If you're a particularly salty sweater (for instance, if you notice salt residue marks on dark-coloured workout clothes).

If you tick one or more of these boxes, you may benefit from using sports drinks that contain added electrolytes (sodium and potassium) during your training, or, if you'd prefer to make your own more natural drink, then fruit juice (such as apple or grape) diluted with about 50% water with ⅛–¼ teaspoon of table salt (ideally iodized) per litre will provide fluid, carbohydrates, potassium (naturally in the fruit) and sodium (from the salt). It's also best not to restrict salt from the diet in your post-exercise nutrition because it can help you retain the ingested fluid, rather than just excreting most of it in the urine.

Now let's discuss carbohydrates. Remember, your body converts the carbs we eat into glycogen for storage in the muscles and liver, and this glycogen is your body's preferred energy source for the moderate-to-high level of activity required in most sports and athletic activities. With the depletion of glycogen stores comes fatigue and reduced power output. As well as this, inadequate carbohydrate as fuel for the brain impairs perceived exertion, motor skills and concentration. But when nutrition is planned well and glycogen stores match the fuel demands of the training session or event, athletes often describe feeling energized, powerful, focused, and of running or cycling as though the wind were behind them.

Before: The main aim for pre-event (or pre-training) nutrition is to provide just the right amount of carbohydrate, in order to keep glycogen stores stocked up in your liver and muscles to keep you fuelled for optimal performance. Glycogen stores are used up each time we exercise, but these stores can be normalized within 24 hours of reduced training and adequate fuel intake (as long as there's no severe muscle damage).[41] So at least one day's rest and plenty of carbs (anywhere between 7–12g/kg/day, e.g. 560–960g a day for an 80kg athlete) will stand you in good stead for shorter-duration activities (up to 60–90 minutes).

Before endurance or high intensity training lasting over 60 minutes, a high-carbohydrate meal 3–4 hours before the training session or event has been shown in numerous studies to improve endurance, power output, interval-style performance (as is common in many team sports) and prolong the time to fatigue.[42–45] Glycogen stores in the liver are lower in the morning because they've been used up during our overnight fast, so this meal can replenish liver glycogen and even some muscle glycogen stores, providing us with energy for sustained exercise. A meal in this time window containing carbohydrates ranging from 3–4g per kg of body weight (e.g. 240–320g for an 80kg athlete) has been shown to be most effective.[46] In general, this meal should be low fat, low fibre, and low to moderate protein in order to reduce the chances of gastrointestinal problems and to promote quicker gastric emptying (so the food is less likely to hang around in your stomach for too long).[47]

Eating carbohydrate-rich foods 30–90 minutes before exercise can also improve endurance performance for some athletes, because the ingested carbohydrate can act as an extra fuel source to supplement the muscle and liver glycogen stores during the exercise. Results for this time frame aren't quite as consistent as they are for the 3–4 hour pre-exercise meal, but if you're training or competing in the morning, this may be the most practical option (rather than waking up at 4 a.m. to get a meal in 3–4 hours before a long 8 a.m. training session). For this option, a smaller meal containing approximately 1–2g/kg is a good general guide (e.g. 80–160g for an 80kg athlete). Just be mindful that in some athletes, eating shortly before exercise can cause stomach discomfort, and in some it can lead to a condition known as rebound hypoglycaemia. This is where the insulin response to the ingested carbohydrate causes low blood sugar, and therefore fatigue, usually just in the early stages of exercise.

However, including a protein source in the meal and choosing low glycaemic-index carbohydrates at this time can help prevent rebound hypoglycaemia.[48] See the table below for more information on the glycaemic index.

FOOD	SERVING SIZE	CARBOHYDRATE CONTENT	GLYCAEMIC INDEX*
White rice, cooked	1 cup	53.2	73
Brown rice, cooked	1 cup	45.8	68
White wheat pasta, cooked	1 cup	64.6	49
Whole wheat pasta, cooked	1 cup	59.2	48
Potato, boiled	1 medium	33.4	78
Chickpeas, cooked	1 cup	45.0	28
Lentils, cooked	1 cup	39.9	32
Oatmeal (porridge), cooked	1 cup	31.8	55
Muesli (fruit and nut)	1 cup	66.1	57
Weetabix	2 biscuits	26.0	69
Banana, raw	1 medium	27.0	51 (62 when ripe**)
Apple, raw	1 medium	25.1	36
Orange juice	1 cup	25.8	50
Gatorade	250ml	15.0	78**
Lucozade original	250ml	22.3	95**

* Glycaemic index scores taken from Harvard Health Publishing, https://www.health.harvard.edu/diseases-and-conditions/glycemic-index-and-glycemic-load-for-100-foods.

** Oregon State University, https://extension.oregonstate.edu/sites/default/files/documents/1/glycemicindex.pdf.

The glycaemic index (GI) value assigned to foods indicates how quickly those foods can cause increases in blood sugar (glucose) levels. Foods with a high GI value release glucose into the bloodstream rapidly, while foods with a low score tend to release glucose more slowly and steadily. In general, I don't encourage clients to pay too much attention to GI scores, because meals nearly always contain several different food groups (e.g. rice, lentils and vegetables), making it more difficult to work out, and because balanced meals usually lead to a steady blood glucose response anyway.[49] However, understanding GI values can be useful when planning pre-event meals, because consuming low GI foods has been shown to help prevent rebound hypoglycaemia for those who are susceptible, and a recent meta-analysis shows it can also be beneficial for endurance performance.[50]

In general, GI scores are considered:

- 55 or lower: low

- 56–69: medium

- 70 or above: high

Let's take two examples:

A 100kg rugby player eating breakfast an hour before a morning game or long training session could benefit from eating 1–2g of carbohydrates per kg of body weight, i.e. 1–200g. This could be achieved with a breakfast of 2 cups of fruit and nut muesli with a banana (approx. 160g of carbs). These foods have a low to medium GI value, so would likely help avoid rebound hypoglycaemia if the athlete was prone to it.

A 60kg cyclist eating a meal 3–4 hours before an afternoon

race or training session should look to eat 3–4g of carbohydrates per kg of body weight, i.e. 180–240g. This meal might consist of 2 cups of cooked white rice, a cup of lentils, a banana, and a glass of orange juice (approx. 200g of carbs).

During: depending on the type of exercise, its duration, and its intensity, carbohydrate intake during exercise can also provide significant benefits to performance. In general, it's not necessary or beneficial to consume carbohydrates during exercise that lasts around 60 minutes or less. With that being said, for exercise that lasts around one hour, there is evidence that just the sensation of carbohydrates in the mouth, even when not swallowed, can stimulate parts of the brain that enhance feelings of wellbeing and have been shown to increase self-selected work output – improving performance by a few per cent.[51, 52]

However, the most significant benefits of nutrition during exercise are seen in longer duration endurance or high intensity 'stop and start' sports (e.g. rugby, football, hockey, basketball and racquet sports) lasting more than 60–90 minutes.[53] In this instance, an intake of 30–60g of carbohydrates per hour during the exercise has been shown to significantly improve performance, especially in the latter stages of exercise when glycogen stores are placed under stress. For the best results, consume carbohydrates at regular intervals, beginning shortly after you start the exercise, and focus on high GI foods. This could be achieved through eating 1–2 bananas (approx. 27–54g of carbs), a sports drink, or a combination of the two may be more practical.

For ultra-distance exercise, lasting over 2.5 hours, there's additional evidence that even higher intakes of carbohydrates – up to 90g per hour during exercise – is associated with improved performance. A previous theory was that muscle was only able to take up and use a maximum of around 1g of carbohydrate per minute (60g per hour) regardless of body size. However, the latest research suggests that we can absorb and oxidize much more if the carbohydrates are comprised of more than one different sugar (i.e. glucose, fructose and sucrose).[54] The good news is that fruits and fruit juices are naturally made up of a variety of sugars – see the chart below – so consuming these will help you to absorb the high amount of carbohydrates, up to 90g per hour, needed to optimally sustain you for ultra-distance events. Sports drinks and gels that are made up of mixed sugar sources (e.g. glucose/fructose mixtures) can be helpful too – gels can be particularly light and practical to carry if you have an opportunity to consume these with water (i.e. regular water stations during a race).

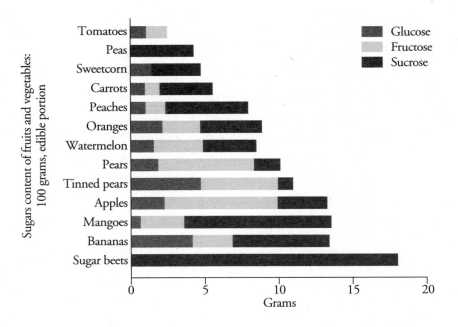

Source: Canadian Sugar Institute (2020)[55]

When considering carbohydrate-containing drinks during exercise, the ultimate goal is to absorb the fluid and sugars (and electrolytes if contained) as rapidly as possible, while being mindful to avoid upsetting the stomach. Drinks with too high a sugar content can delay gastric emptying and are slower to be absorbed in the intestine, so can cause intestinal discomfort and sometimes diarrhoea. Research shows that drinks with 6–8% carbohydrate by volume, ideally with mixed sources (e.g. glucose and fructose) are generally emptied quickly from the stomach, are well absorbed, and can help with hydration. Most sports drinks like Gatorade and Powerade fit the bill nicely. Be mindful, though, that some commercial energy drinks and fizzy drinks are much more concentrated and so can cause stomach upset if used during exercise. Likewise, many fruit juices have much more than 8% carbohydrates. Apple juice, for example, typically contains 11–12% carbohydrate, and so would benefit from being diluted with water to be better tolerated and absorbed if taken during exercise. Likewise, sports gels and easily digested solid foods like fruit should always be consumed with plenty of water for the same reasons.

As with any fuelling strategies, it's always a good idea to practise them during training first to figure out what works best for you, taking into account your personal food preferences and gut comfort. You might also need to consider what's most practical for the rules and nature of your sport (e.g. whether solid food is allowed during match play, what's easiest to carry on a bike, etc).

After: It's recommended that athletes consume a mixed meal after exercise containing carbohydrates, protein and fat, alongside plenty of fluids. One of the key goals of the post-exercise meal (alongside stimulating muscle protein synthesis and rehydrating) is to replenish glycogen stores. The rate of glycogen resynthesis — how fast your body converts the carbohydrates you eat into glycogen for storage in the muscles and liver — is only about 5% per hour.[56] So an early intake of carbohydrates in the recovery period is useful in maximizing that effective refuelling time. This is especially important when there is another bout of exercise anticipated the same day or in successive days.

Carbohydrate loading

In the lead-up to an important endurance event or a high intensity 'stop and go' sporting match lasting more than 90 minutes, it's possible to elevate glycogen stores to even higher than normal levels, which can significantly improve performance, through a process called carbohydrate loading.[57] Original protocols involved first depleting glycogen stores through an exhaustive bout of exercise followed by a very low carbohydrate diet for 3 days, and then 3 days of a high carbohydrate diet. This was found to be effective at achieving 'super-compensation' of muscle glycogen stores, above those found even on a regular high-carbohydrate diet. But it's no longer recommended because of the negative side-effects during the low carbohydrate phase, such as weakness, irritability, food cravings and increased susceptibility to infection: it's just not worth the discomfort and increased risk of illness, especially before an important event.

Evidence shows that the 'super-compensation' of glycogen stores can still be achieved without the prior depletion stage.[58, 59] So current protocols instead suggest omitting the depletion stage, but tapering your training and consuming a very high carbohydrate diet for up to 3 days before competition. The carbohydrate intake during this time can be as high as 70% of total calories, or anywhere between 7–12g per kg of body weight a day, i.e. 560–960g of carbohydrate per day for an athlete weighing 80kg. This takes some effort, and is much more than simply having a big bowl of pasta the night before a race (as many people believe carbohydrate loading to be). Fat and protein intake will likely have to be lowered during this time to ensure overall caloric intake isn't in surplus, and some athletes will benefit from emphasizing non whole grain options to prevent higher than usual fibre intakes.

ERGOGENIC AIDS FOR PERFORMANCE

Now you know how best to fuel your body, and how to time your nutrition around competitions and key training sessions to achieve peak performance. These strategies alone can help you make dramatic progress in your sport or activity. But is there anything else we can be doing to give us an edge over the competition?

This is where, for some, ergogenic aids can come in. These are techniques or substances used for the purposes of enhancing performance, and can range from natural whole foods, to banned illegal drugs. There are countless non-nutrition ergogenic aids too, ranging from sport-specific techniques like shaving legs and using a swimming cap to reduce drag in the water for swimmers, to general lifestyle adjustments such as improving the quantity/quality of your sleep, which, as we'll discuss in the next chapter, can serve as a potent performance enhancer.

However, in this section, we'll just look at the nutritional factors and supplements that could improve performance, with a focus on those that may be of particular interest to plant-based athletes. We've already covered some of these, such as carbohydrate timing for sports, and getting plenty of dietary flavanols and antioxidants through a balanced plant-based diet, which can reduce muscle fatigue and increase endurance capacity.

But many athletes, perhaps because of their inherently competitive nature, look for other ways, such as dietary supplements, to gain that competitive edge. And supplements can indeed be a legitimate part of an elite athlete's preparation, when used appropriately and responsibly. There are countless examples in sporting history where the difference between first and second place comes down to hundredths of a second, or where winning a sprint to the ball in the final stages of a match can help clinch a game. It's these instances in particular where ergogenic aids can make all the difference.

However, most statements about the health or performance enhancing effects on the labels of many products are not backed by clear scientific evidence. Because of this, institutions such as the Australian Institute of Sport and the American College of Sports Medicine have created systems to classify supplements according to their effects on performance based on confirmed scientific evidence.[60, 61] The supplements covered in this chapter are the ones classed with the highest level of evidence to improve performance when taken in the appropriate amounts and in the right setting.

I like to think of ergogenic supplements as the icing on the cake: the foundations are far more important, so it's critical to get the basics right first before fine-tuning the smaller details. There are no shortcuts when it comes to maximizing your performance and you can't expect supplements to replace a healthy balanced diet and lifestyle – you have to put in the groundwork first before building up to the more intricate details. So I like to encourage my clients to consider the following questions before evaluating whether or not a supplement might be beneficial:

- Do you eat enough but not excessive amounts of energy to support your level of training?
- Is your plant-based diet varied, balanced, and based mostly around whole plant foods?
- Do you take appropriate steps to ensure you get sufficient amounts of the key nutrients for vegans (i.e. those covered in Chapter 5)?
- Do you drink enough water to keep properly hydrated throughout the day and during your training?
- Do you take all steps to improve the quality and quantity of your sleep?
- Have you considered your carbohydrate timing around your training and events?
- Do you follow optimal training principles as advised by a coach or trainer?

If you answer no to any of these questions, I would first encourage you to go back to basics, and make sure each of these areas is fully covered before considering whether to use ergogenic supplements. If you answered yes to all of the questions, and if you feel a further slight enhancement would benefit at the level you compete at, then they may be worth considering.

This is by no means an exhaustive list of the available supplements, but a handful chosen either because there's sufficient evidence to support their benefits to athletes in general, or because plant-based athletes specifically tend to take in smaller amounts of these substances naturally through the diet. This is in no way an endorsement of their use, but an effort to provide information on their potential benefits and risks based on the latest and most robust research, in order for you to decide for yourself whether or not they're appropriate for you.

Caffeine

Caffeine is the most widely consumed psychoactive drug in the world, because in most cultures it's widely accepted and easily accessible.[62] Here in the UK we consume an average of 70 million cups of coffee a day, but caffeine is also found in tea and chocolate, and is often added to fizzy drinks, sports drinks, bars and gels, and certain medications.

There's a wealth of research on the performance effects of caffeine. In fact, so much research has been done that it's been possible to conduct numerous meta-analyses of individual studies, and a recent umbrella review to assess 21 of these published meta-analyses (an analysis of meta-analyses – research doesn't get much better than that!). It showed the evidence is that caffeine does indeed exert a significant ergogenic effect on muscle endurance, muscle strength, anaerobic power and aerobic endurance.[63]

There are several suggested mechanisms by which caffeine's ergogenic effects come about, but a key one is thought to be by stimulating the central nervous system. It does this by blocking a chemical called adenosine, which builds up in the brain throughout the day and has a negative effect on neurotransmission, wakefulness, and pain perception. As such, caffeine can reduce fatigue, dampen pain reception, blunt our perception of effort, and improve alertness and concentration.[64, 65] All this leads to significant improved performance, in most people. Recent research shows that, contrary to popular belief, caffeine consumed even at moderately high intakes does not lead to dehydration during exercise[66] and habitual caffeine intake doesn't seem to affect its short-term ergogenic properties.[67]

So how much caffeine, and when, should we consume to benefit from this ergogenic effect? The answers to these questions are not clear-cut, and should be tailored to the individual. The majority of the studies in the large umbrella review mentioned above provided the caffeine supplementation one hour before exercise, which seems to be an effective time window. Most also used a large single dose of caffeine at between 3–6mg/kg of bodyweight. For example, a 70kg athlete would have taken between 210–420mg of caffeine. However, there's a growing body of evidence to show that lower doses, under 3mg/kg of bodyweight, can still have a significant ergogenic effect.[68] This could be achieved simply through drinking 1–2 cups of strong coffee.

To weigh up whether caffeine might be appropriate for you, it's important to consider the potential risks and side-effects. Some people hardly notice a difference after several strong coffees, whereas others (me included!) are highly sensitive to caffeine, and even low amounts can cause

FOOD OR DRINK	SERVING SIZE	TYPICAL CAFFEINE CONTENT (mg)
Coffee, brewed from grounds*	240ml (1 cup)	96
Coffee, instant*	Dry weight 0.9g (1 tsp)	28
Coffee, espresso*	60ml (1 espresso cup)	127
Breakfast tea, brewed 5 minutes†	170ml (6oz)	25
Breakfast tea, brewed 3 minutes†	170ml (6oz)	22
Green tea, brewed 3 minutes†	170ml (6oz)	27–46
Dark chocolate, 70–85% cocoa solids*	28g (1oz)	23
Coca Cola, original**	330ml (1 can)	32
Coca Cola, diet**	330ml (1 can)	42
Red Bull, regular**	250ml (1 can)	80
Lucozade, original**	380ml (1 bottle)	46
Pro Plus**	1 tablet	50

* Data from USDA FoodData Central https://fdc.nal.usda.gov and individual brand nutrition information.

** Selected manufacturers.

† https://www.researchgate.net/publication/23471909_Caffeine_Content_of_Brewed_Teas.

anxiousness and restlessness, and in some can lead to headaches and nausea. This difference in caffeine metabolism is mostly genetic – if you're in the latter group, then it may be best to stick to lower intakes (<3mg/kg body weight) or eschew caffeine altogether, as those side-effects may offset any improvements in performance and detract from the enjoyment of the sport or training. You should also bear in mind how caffeine can impact sleep, and that tea and coffee can affect the absorption of certain minerals, especially iron, as we discussed in Chapter 5.

Finally, you should also check with your sport's governing body whether caffeine is permitted, and at what doses. For example, although the International Olympic Committee removed caffeine from its list of restricted substances in 2004, it's still banned by the National Collegiate Athletic Association (NCAA) at very high concentrations corresponding to ingesting around 500mg.

Creatine

Creatine is a natural organic compound, made in the body, primarily by the liver and kidneys. It's mostly found in the skeletal muscles, where it exists in the forms of free creatine, and creatine phosphate, which acts as an important storage form of energy – it facilitates the recycling of ATP, which can be thought of as the energy currency of our cells.

The body produces creatine using the amino acids glycine, arginine and methionine. So, as long as you're getting enough of these amino acids in your diet, which as we discussed in Chapter 6 is highly likely, you'll be making sufficient amounts of creatine for healthy functioning yourself. Still, meat-eaters get some additional creatine through the diet (an average of around 2g per day[69]), which makes sense, given that creatine is found primarily in muscle tissue – including that of other animals. By comparison, the dietary intake of creatine in vegans is negligible. This is why lower concentrations of creatine are often found in the blood and skeletal muscle of those on a plant-based diet.[70]

There's been a considerable amount of research conducted on creatine supplementation over the last two decades. Meta-analyses show that taken in supplement form, creatine can provide benefits in two ways: first, by significantly increasing muscle creatine stores, it can improve performance in high-intensity, short-duration exercises (such as weight training and the interval-style anaerobic power required in many team sports).[72-74] Second, supplementation has also been shown to improve adaptations to training, leading to greater gains in lean muscle mass, strength, and power over time.[75] This is likely through several specific mechanisms that favour an anabolic (muscle building) environment, as well as due to the higher metabolic demand created by the more intensely per-formed training sessions.[76]

Because vegans and vegetarians tend to have lower baseline muscle creatine levels, evidence shows that those on a plant-based diet respond even better to creatine supplementation than omnivores. For instance, a study looking at vegetarian and non-vegetarian responses to creatine supplementation while training showed that, as expected, all participants taking creatine had greater increases in creatine stores, muscle strength, and whole-body muscle mass than those in the placebo groups. But, interestingly, the vegetarian sub-group supplementing with creatine had a significantly greater increase in creatine stores, whole-body muscle mass, and total work performance than the non-vegetarians who also took creatine.[77] So it's often suggested that plant-based ath-letes taking part in strength training or sports with explosive movements can benefit the most from regular or periodic creatine supplementation.

What about dosage and timings? A commonly used pro-tocol is to follow a high intake (20–30g a day) during a 'loading' phase for about a week, followed by a lower ongoing 'maintenance' dose of 3–5g a day. The loading phase is designed to quickly saturate creatine stores in skeletal muscle, and once saturated, the lower 3–5g daily intake can maintain these levels. The loading phase can be omitted, and a daily intake of 3–5g a day will also lead to the same increases in muscle creatine levels over time, but it may just take a little longer (3–4 weeks) to maximize your stores.[78]

Timings-wise, it doesn't seem too important. Some research shows that consuming it shortly after resistance training is slightly more beneficial for increasing muscle mass compared to supplementation immediately before training.[79–81] Likely to be of greater importance would be consuming creatine at the same time as carbohydrate and/or protein sources, as this seems to promote uptake into skeletal muscle by around 25% thanks to the body's insulin response.[82]

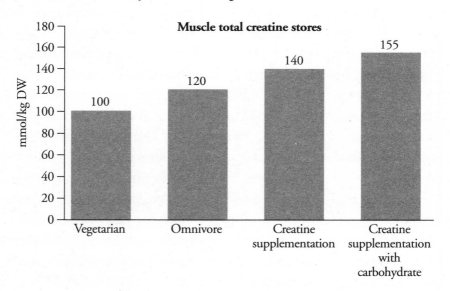

Source: Kreider & Jung (2011)[71]

Creatine's not screened for or banned by the World Doping Agency, the International Olympic Committee, or the NCAA. It's now widely used among recreational, amateur and professional athletes, for example an estimated 37% of English professional footballers say they use creatine.[83, 84] A large amount of evidence shows that supplementing appropriately is safe both in the short and long term (up to 5 years). In fact, the International Society of Sports Nutrition (ISSN) released their official position stating that on the mass of evidence, creatine supplementation is not only safe, but has been reported to have a number of therapeutic effects.[85] For instance, in a study specifically designed to assess its safety, American football players supplemented with creatine for 21 months were assessed using 69 health markers, including kidney function, muscle and liver enzymes, metabolic markers, electrolytes and blood lipids. Those supplementing had no difference in risk factors for any of the health markers.[86] In fact, creatine users experienced less incidence of cramping, heat illness/dehydration, muscle strains and total injuries than those not taking creatine.[87]

It should be mentioned that most of the studies on creatine use are conducted in adults. There's evidence to suggest that it's also safe in adolescent athletes, but still, if you're under 18 years, the ISSN recommend you should only consider creatine use if you a) are involved in serious/competitive supervised training; b) are already consuming a well-balanced and performance-enhancing diet; c) are knowledgeable about appropriate use of creatine; and d) do not exceed recommended dosages. To be honest, these are the prerequisites I would look for in adult use anyway. Also, if you're an endurance athlete, taking creatine will not provide any beneficial effects on aerobic performance.[88] In fact the opposite may be true – it can be detrimental in events where body mass must be moved against gravity (such as jumping athletic events) or when a specific body mass needs to be reached.[89]

Creatine monohydrate is the most extensively studied and clinically effective form of creatine, so if you do choose to try creatine, this would be the safest option. Look for this in its pure form, rather than mixed with a variety of other ingredients as is sometimes found in commercial sports products. There are several brands certified as vegan, and some that are third-party tested for quality and purity, which is advised.

Beetroot juice

We discussed earlier in the chapter how higher intake of dietary nitrates, as is common in plant-based diets, is one of the reasons why vegans regularly see improvements in their performance. Research shows that habitual intake of dietary nitrates, through eating plenty of nitrate-rich vegetables, including beetroot and green leafy vegetables like rocket, lettuce, spinach and cress, is an easy strategy to optimize performance.[90] The performance-enhancing effects have also been shown to increase over time,[91] great news for vegans who regularly eat plenty of these nitrate-rich green leafy vegetables.

They're worth a mention in this chapter too, because dietary nitrates can also serve as a more immediate, acute ergogenic aid when consumed before exercise. The reason this section is labelled 'beetroot juice' rather than 'nitrates' is because beetroot juice is a particularly concentrated, natural form of nitrates and as such has been used in much of the research into the ergogenic effects of nitrates. There's also evidence that beetroot juice is more effective than supplementation in the form of sodium nitrate in improving the energy efficiency of exercise,[92] and many athletes feel more comfortable using natural whole foods rather than man-made supplements where possible.

In terms of performance enhancement, there are substantial amounts of evidence to show the benefits of beetroot juice supplementation. A systematic review analysed 23 studies and concluded that its use as a supplement can improve cardiorespiratory endurance in athletes by increasing exercise efficiency, which improves performance at various distances. It can also increase the time to exhaustion and may improve performance at anaerobic threshold intensities and maximal oxygen uptake.[93] Two other systematic reviews indicate that nitrates and beetroot juice significantly reduce the oxygen cost of submaximal exercise and improve performance during high-intensity endurance exercise.[94, 95]

We already know that the nitrates in beetroot juice achieve these benefits by increasing levels of nitric oxide, an important signalling molecule which can help improve blood flow to the muscles during exercise. But this nitric oxide can also promote oxygen and glucose transfer into the muscle, improve the efficiency of mitochondrial function (the mitochondria are the energy-producing 'powerhouses' within our cells), and enhance the muscle contraction and relaxation processes.[96, 97] All of this translates into tangible results: in trained cyclists, supplementing with beetroot juice improved cycle times by 1–3% in tests ranging from 4–80 kilometres;[98] in runners, time to exhaustion at high-intensity paces was increased by 15%;[99] a 500m kayaking time trial performance was improved by 1.7%;[100] and a 3.5% improvement was seen in sprint performance during interval training designed to reflect the dynamic work profile of team sport play.[101] Results have even been seen in weight training, with participants able to add seven additional bench press repetitions over three sets at 60% of their 1-rep max compared to a placebo-controlled group.[102]

There are, however, some studies assessing beetroot juice supplementation which don't show a significant benefit. There could be many reasons why that's the case, including age and diet of the participant, and the exercise conditions. However, there appear to be two key reasons why effects aren't shown in certain studies: firstly, the ergogenic effects seem to be less obvious in highly trained athletes – while elite athletes seem to benefit a little from beetroot juice, a meta-analysis shows that the largest effects have been shown in healthy, recreationally active participants.[103] The second reason could be down to timing: several studies have left just 60–90 minutes between supplementation and exercise, while it's thought that the ergogenic effects are seen around 2.5–3 hours after supplementation.[104]

What about dosage – how much beetroot juice should we have if we want to benefit from its performance-enhancing properties? The majority of studies show ergogenic effects with a dose of around 6–8mmol (370–500mg) of nitrate. Although the amount of nitrate in beetroot juice can vary considerably, in general this can be achieved with around 1–2 cups.[105] Beetroot juice concentrate 'shots' are also available, which may be more convenient for travelling, etc. It's also possible that highly trained athletes might require a slightly higher dose – for example, the study conducted in elite kayakers above showed ergogenic effects at around 600mg of nitrates but results didn't improve at 300mg.[106] Even these levels are significantly less than the amount that leads to toxicity.[107]

Beetroots are incredibly healthy – not only are they rich in nitrates but the pigments that give them their dark red colour, called betalains, have powerful antioxidant properties. These pigments can, however, cause red or pink urine. This condition, known as beeturia, is harmless but can be startling if you don't expect it. Because the concentrated source of nitrates can help to lower blood pressure, which is a good thing for many people, it's advised not to drink beetroot juice regularly if you already have low blood pressure. Also bear in mind that beetroots are a source of oxalates, which as we covered in Chapter 5 can impact the absorption of some minerals, particularly calcium. Beetroot juice can also cause stomach upset or diarrhoea in some people – so as with any new dietary approach, if you plan to try it as an ergogenic aid, experiment during training and don't try new things during key events.

Beta-alanine and sodium bicarbonate

These final two ergogenic aids work through different mechanisms but both have the same goal: to help dampen the build-up of acid in the muscles during high-intensity exercise. An acidic environment in the muscle impairs performance and is one of many factors that contribute to the onset of muscle fatigue. Many of you will be all too familiar with that feeling during high-intensity exercise when our muscles feel like they're on fire! These ergogenic aids certainly won't take away that sensation, but may help to eke out a little extra effort just at the key moment when our muscles feel as though they're about to fail, specifically during high-intensity events lasting from around one up to a few minutes.

You can see from the graph on page 174 that during maximal effort within this time frame, the body is relying heavily on anaerobic glycolysis for energy. This means that after the muscle cells' immediate energy currency stores (ATP and creatine) have been depleted, the body is reliant on breaking down glucose for energy without the use of oxygen, and it's this process that results in an acidic environment in the muscles and results in that often excruciating burning sensation! Shortly after this time, the body uses oxygen to break down glucose for its main source of energy, which is key for endurance exercise and shown on the graph as the aerobic system. However, if further bursts of high-intensity movement are required during endurance exercise (e.g. as is required during many team sports, or for a longer race 'sprint finish'), then the anaerobic system will likely take over as the dominant energy source again. So the extra ability to buffer the acidity can help improve performance in both high-intensity exercise and the capacity of high-intensity sprints during endurance exercise.

Beta-alanine is a non-essential amino acid, and is used by the body to make carnosine, which acts in the skeletal

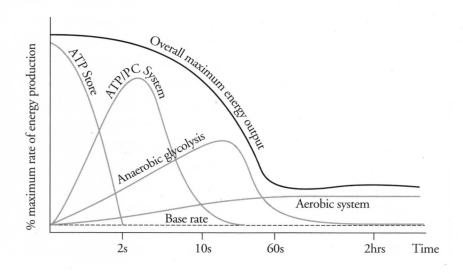

muscles to reduce that acid accumulation during exercise. Supplementing with beta-alanine increases muscle carnosine content (by up to 80% of resting levels) and can provide small yet significant performance benefits of around 2–3% in exercise tests. Specifically, results from two meta-analyses showed improvements in performance of continuous or intermittent high-intensity exercise lasting between 30 seconds and 10 minutes.[108, 109] Because some studies show that muscle carnosine levels tend to be lower in vegans and vegetarians,[110, 111] beta-alanine supplementation could result in even greater performance improvements for plant-based athletes.[112]

The general protocol for beta-alanine supplementation is 3–6g a day, taken for a minimum of 2–4 weeks, but with continued improvements in muscle carnosine stores when taken for 10–12 weeks. Dosing strategies of taking smaller amounts split over the course of the day (such as 1g every 3–4 hours) are popular because this minimizes the risk of side-effects, which can range from itchiness and skin rashes to temporary 'tingling' of the skin, known as paraesthesia.[113] Beta-alanine consumption may also be a little less effective in highly trained athletes, because they already have enhanced acid buffering capacity – studies show smaller improvements in performance in well-trained athletes of between 0.2–1.3%.[114, 115] But small percentages like these can certainly be meaningful, perhaps even pivotal, in the context of elite competition.

Sodium bicarbonate (known as bicarbonate of soda, or simply baking soda) also works to buffer the build-up of acid during high-intensity exercise, but works in a different way to beta-alanine (or more precisely carnosine): rather than working within the muscle cells, it augments the ability of the extracellular fluid (the fluid that bathes our muscle cells) to draw out excess acid from the exercising muscle cells.

Performance enhancements of around 2% have been documented. As with beta-alanine, the effects seem to be most prominent for exercise lasting up to a few minutes.[116] That being said, significant performance benefits are also seen with higher numbers of repeated sprint bouts, as is often required in team sports.[117]

Supplementation is just taken before exercise (rather than on an ongoing basis as with beta-alanine) and involves consuming 0.2–0.4g per kilogram of body weight (i.e. 16–32g for an 80kg athlete). Supplements usually come in the form of capsules or in a fluid solution and are taken 1–2 hours before exercise. The main issue with sodium bicarbonate supplementation is that gastrointestinal (GI) upset is a common side-effect, and may even completely negate any performance benefits in some people. A strategy to minimize GI upset includes consuming the sodium bicarbonate alongside a small carbohydrate-containing meal or splitting the dose into several smaller doses over the course of 30–60 minutes.[118, 119] If you do intend to try sodium bicarbonate, it's a prime example of the importance of testing it out during training – if you are affected by GI problems, it's better to find out during a training session than write off an important competition performance!

As you've seen in this chapter, the potential of a plant-based diet to enhance performance shouldn't be underestimated. Numerous nutrients that are found in higher abundance in whole plant foods – such as a huge range of antioxidants, dietary flavanols, and nitrates – can produce powerful effects within the body that can boost performance in a range of sporting disciplines. You're also now equipped with the knowledge of how to further augment these effects with proven fuelling strategies and nutrition timing tips to get the most out of your training. Then, the icing on the cake could be the appropriate use of certain ergogenic aids, which can take your performance to the next level. Before we go on to turn all the theory into practice by customizing our own meal plans, we'll spend some time considering some other lifestyle factors that can be equally important for both protecting health and improving performance.

CHAPTER 8

OTHER IMPORTANT LIFESTYLE HABITS FOR HEALTH AND PERFORMANCE

My area of expertise is nutrition. I just love how the science provides us with evidence which we can apply to achieve profound effects on both our health and our performance. Putting the theory into practice and watching clients truly thrive and out-perform their competition while eating a plant-based diet is my biggest motivation. But there are several other lifestyle factors that are so closely and intricately intertwined with nutrition, health and performance that I feel they're far too important not to mention. They go hand-in-hand, and together they lay the foundations for great achievements.

Picture the scenario – a sportsperson is doing everything right with their training. In fact they're making sacrifices to make sure they're training harder than the rest of the competition. They're doing everything to optimize their nutrition: getting all the key nutrients, timing carbohydrates to fuel the workouts, keeping hydrated, eating right to maximize muscle protein synthesis, and possibly even using some ergogenic aids to boost performance in training and match play. But if this athlete has poor sleep habits and isn't managing their stress as well as they could, as we'll see in this chapter, there's clear evidence showing that making progress will be much, much harder, from both a psychological and a physiological aspect. With so much effort going into the training and nutrition, it seems a real shame that such basic, fundamental lifestyle factors are holding them back.

So I'd like to use the following pages as an opportunity to get you thinking about these other lifestyle factors – because the vast majority of people go through life without giving these parts much thought at all. If we can at least bring them into our consciousness and make some efforts to improve them, when done alongside our nutrition and training, that's when truly astonishing results start to happen in terms of our health, energy, happiness, and performance.

SLEEP

Cast your mind back to the last time you got a really good night's uninterrupted sleep, and woke up feeling truly rested, energized and invigorated. Was it last weekend? Last month? Last year? Getting enough sleep is critical for our health, wellbeing and performance, yet studies show that most people in the UK, and in many other Western nations, get less than the 8 hours a night recommended for adults by the World Health Organization. In fact, a recent poll revealed that in Britain, only a small minority – 1 in 5 people – are getting at least 8 hours' sleep a night.[1]

I think we can all agree that a good night's sleep feels great. But many aspects are out of our control, such as noise outside our home, long work hours or shift patterns, other health issues, having babies or children (with a young toddler, this one resonates with me!), or other commitments. So this section isn't about setting specific goals with your sleep, as everyone's circumstances are different, and certain goals just might not be realistic for some people. It's more about understanding the importance of sleep for our health, well-being and performance, because most people aren't aware of just how valuable it is and therefore don't prioritize their sleep. We'll also look at some simple proven ways we can promote healthy sleep, which can result in stark improvements in terms of energy, health, happiness, and progress with your training.

Researchers have made huge advances in understanding how sleep can impact our health. In fact, so much research has been done that it's been possible to conduct several large meta-analyses to reveal some fascinating (albeit morbid) discoveries about out how sleep can impact some of the most major and prevalent diseases in the West. These meta-analyses show that inadequate or poor-quality sleep is associated with significantly increased risk of high blood pressure, cardiovascular disease, Alzheimer's disease, cancer, diabetes and weight gain.[2-8] In fact, one large meta-analysis showed that sleeping too little at night significantly increases the risk of early death.[9, 10] In these studies, inadequate sleep was usually classified as under 7 hours – which is the amount nearly half of us in the UK usually get.

The mechanisms linking lack of sleep with all these diseases are complex, inter-related, and still not yet fully understood. But we do know that many of the responses associated with sleep deprivation result from over-activation of the sympathetic nervous system, which is responsible for the body's ability to deal with danger (otherwise known as the 'flight or fight' response). The sympathetic nervous system regulates almost every organ function in the body: it dilates pupils, raises heart rate and blood pressure, decreases gut movement, promotes systemic inflammation, and directs blood to our muscles, as if the body were preparing to endure a physical attack. But when overstimulated chronically (as insufficient sleep seems to promote), the ongoing strain put on the body manifests in a whole host of health issues. For instance, the persistently elevated heart rate and blood pressure puts added force on our artery walls, making them more vulnerable to the damage that leads to cardiovascular diseases such as heart attack and stroke. We also know that sleep disturbances cause increases in key markers of systemic inflammation.[11] When experienced over a long duration, as we saw in Chapter 3, this is an underlying mechanism behind most diseases, ranging from diabetes to cancer.

Another area where there's been a lot of research is how sleep can affect appetite and weight gain, with several meta-analyses linking chronic short sleep with weight gain and obesity.[12–14] Why does this happen? Sleep loss has been shown to increase levels of the hormone ghrelin – known as the hunger hormone, which drives our appetite.[15] As if that weren't bad enough, sleep loss also decreases levels of leptin, a hormone whose job is to let us know we're full when we've eaten.[16] Adding to this, there also seems to be a greater firing up of the neuronal reward pathways of the brain in response to unhealthy food compared to healthy food after a period of restricted sleep.[17] All this leads to unrelenting food cravings that even the strongest-willed athlete finds hard to resist.

Insufficient sleep can also significantly impact our mental health, with strong links with risk of depression and anxiety.[18, 19] The cause of this link can work in both directions: there's evidence that lack of sleep can be a contributing factor to mental health problems, while anxiety and depression can both cause sleep disturbances.[20] The result can be a self-perpetuating cycle: lack of sleep makes us feel more anxious/depressed, which in turn makes it harder to sleep.

At the other end of the spectrum, studies show that sleeping well can improve what's known as positive affect – a state of pleasurable engagement with the environment that elicits feelings such as happiness, joy, excitement, enthusiasm and contentment.[21, 22] I believe I can safely say that these are all emotions we'd like to feel more of the time!

The quantity and quality of sleep can significantly impact sports and exercise performance too – through both psychological and physiological aspects. This may be especially important to high-level athletes because there's evidence that many elite athletes don't sleep as well as their non-athletic counterparts,[23] likely due to large training volumes, early morning training, the added stresses of competitions/events, and sometimes travel times and jetlag for competitions.[24, 25]

Let's look first at how good sleep can give you the mental edge. Getting enough sleep has been shown in meta-analyses to improve a variety of cognitive functions, ranging from attention, processing speed, learning, decision-making, reaction times, short-term memory and prospective memory (remembering to do something in the future).[26–28] All these aspects are critical in sports settings, and translate into tangible results for athletes and sports teams. For example, serving accuracy was up to 53% higher in tennis players who were able to get sufficient sleep vs those who got a single night of 5 hours' sleep;[29] collegiate basketball players who extended their sleep patterns experienced a 9% improved shooting accuracy;[30] and football players showed a significantly steeper learning curve for the performance of sport-specific tasks like agility tests compared to when they were sleep deprived.[31]

What about physiological impacts of sleep on performance such as strength and aerobic capacity? That too is closely correlated, especially when it comes to endurance performance. For example, distance covered on a 30-minute treadmill test was 7% shorter in subjects after sleep deprivation;[32] while time trials in triathletes were improved by 3% after just 4 days of extended sleep periods.[33] In fact a systematic review of 10 studies showed longer sleep had a positive effect on subsequent performance in a wide range of sports.[34] One of the key mechanisms linking sleep with performance lies in the perceived level of exertion – athletes doing the same level of work seem to find it easier after sleeping better.[35] On top of this, pre-exercise glycogen stores have also been found to be decreased after sleep deprivation, which would counter all the hard work you put in with your fuelling strategies from Chapter 7 to raise glycogen stores.[36]

We've looked mostly at the effects of short-term sleep duration/quality on performance, but what about the long-term effects? As we know from Chapter 6, one of the holy grails of sports and exercise nutrition is promoting muscle protein synthesis (MPS). But sleep is a non-nutritional approach which is also extremely valuable. Just one night of sleep deprivation has been shown to increase levels of the stress hormone cortisol, and reduce testosterone levels, and this hormonal shift results in significantly lower rates of MPS.[37] Long-term studies are sparse, but population-based studies on shift-workers who experience altered sleep patterns experience negative changes in skeletal muscle health.[38] So while short-term sleep deprivation seems to mostly impact endurance-based performance, long-term sleep loss is likely to have severe consequences on MPS and resulting performance in power/strength-based activities too.

There's one more important aspect regarding sleep's effects on performance worth discussing here: time out due to injury or illness. While you might not at first see the connection between your sleep and risk of injury, there's evidence that impaired or decreased sleep can in fact significantly increase risk. For instance, in a study of high school athletes, those who slept under 8 hours a night were 70% more likely to pick up an injury than those who slept more than 8 hours.[39] In addition, a study in almost 500 athletes from 16 different team and individual sports showed that decreased sleep volume increased risk of injury by 46% independently of training load and intensity.[40] It's thought that the resulting impairments in reaction time, cognitive function and fatigue after sleep deprivation could predispose the athletes to acute injury. Sleep loss is also immunosuppressive and in particular increases susceptibility to upper respiratory tract infections,[41, 42] which is something else that can set back your training or dash dreams of setting a personal best in competition.

Tips for better sleep

Like I said at the start of this section, the aim is to raise awareness of the importance of sleep and how it can have a profound effect on your health and performance. If you can improve the quantity or quality of your sleep even just a little,

you could see drastic improvements in your health and performance. Here are 10 tips to better sleep that could help you
achieve just that:*

1. **Stick to a sleep schedule of the same bedtime
   and wake-up time, even on the weekends.**
   Having different sleep/wake times on the weekends
   is known as social jetlag and can significantly
   impair sleep quality during the week.[43]
2. **Practise a relaxing bedtime ritual.** A relaxing
   routine activity right before bedtime, conducted
   away from bright lights, helps separate your sleep
   time from activities that can cause excitement,
   stress or anxiety, which can make it more difficult
   to fall asleep, get sound and deep sleep, or remain
   asleep. Try reading or practising mindfulness before
   bed rather than using electronic devices to help
   wind down.
3. **If you have trouble sleeping, avoid naps,
   especially in the afternoon.** Power napping may
   help you get through the day, but if you find that
   you can't fall asleep at bedtime, eliminating even
   short catnaps may help.
4. **Exercise daily.** Even 30 minutes of light exercise
   like hiking or cycling can significantly improve your
   sleep. Try not to exercise too late in the day, as it
   can take some time for your adrenaline to return to
   baseline levels.

* These tips are adapted from the National Sleep Foundation: https://www.
sleepfoundation.org/articles/healthy-sleep-tips.

5. **Evaluate your room.** Design your sleep environment to establish the conditions you need for healthy sleep. Your bedroom should be cool – around 16–19°C (60–67°F). Your bedroom should also be free from any noise that can disturb your sleep and ideally kept tidy to help build a relaxing environment without distractions. Finally, your bedroom should be free from any light. Consider using blackout curtains, eye shades, ear plugs, and 'white noise' machines or fans to create ambient sound.

6. **Sleep on a comfortable mattress and pillows.** Make sure your mattress is comfortable and supportive, and hasn't exceeded its life expectancy. Have comfortable pillows and make the room attractive and inviting for sleep but also free of allergens that might affect you.

7. **Use light to help manage your body clock.** Daylight is critical for regulating your sleep patterns – expose yourself to sunlight in the mornings and turn down the lights before bedtime. This will keep your circadian rhythms in check. Blue light emitted from many screens (including smartphones, tablets, computers and laptops) can suppress melatonin, the hormone that regulates the sleep/wake cycle, so try not to use screens for an hour or so before bed (this ties in nicely with tip number 2).

8. **Avoid caffeine and nicotine.** Caffeine is a stimulant and its effects can take up to 8 hours to wear off fully. People often don't make the connection between a cup of coffee late in the afternoon and difficulty sleeping. Be mindful of

caffeine in coffee, teas, colas and sports drinks, and chocolate. Nicotine is also a stimulant which can impair sleep. Smokers also sometimes wake up too early because of nicotine withdrawal.

9. **Avoid alcohol and heavy meals in the evening.** Alcohol may help you relax, but it affects your sleep cycle, keeping you in a lighter sleep and denying you valuable REM sleep.[44] Large meals can also cause indigestion, which can affect sleep, and drinking too much liquid at night can cause frequent awakenings to urinate.

10. **If you can't sleep:** Go into another room and do something relaxing until you feel tired. It is best to take work materials, computers and televisions out of the sleeping environment. Use your bed only for sleep and sex to strengthen the association between bed and sleep. If you associate a particular activity or item with anxiety about sleeping, omit it from your bedtime routine.

If you're still having trouble sleeping, don't hesitate to speak with your doctor or to find a sleep professional. You may also benefit from recording your sleep in a sleep diary to help you better evaluate common patterns or issues you may see with your sleep or sleeping habits.

MOVEMENT

Exercise is another fundamental pillar of health and well-being. The health benefits are countless, and they're closely intertwined with nutrition, sleep, stress and even social relationships. Of course if you're an athlete, you probably already do lots of exercise, which is brilliant. But it's still important to understand just how vital exercise is for our health – both physical and mental – because some studies show that a considerable proportion of athletes dramatically decline their physical activity levels or live sedentary lives after retirement from competitive sports.[45, 46]

Something else that many of my clients are unaware of is the importance of reducing and breaking up long periods of sedentary activities, which is something even elite-level sportspeople can be prone to. So, even if you are already highly active, learning a little more about the impact of movement could bring further benefits to your overall health and performance.

Let's first look at how regular exercise can improve our physical health. The evidence is clear: meta-analyses and systematic reviews have found that increased levels of physical activity are associated with significantly reduced risk of the major diseases in the West: cardiovascular disease (including heart attack and stroke), type 2 diabetes, obesity, several cancers and Alzheimer's disease.[47–52] In fact, exercise helps us live longer – it reduces risk of all-cause mortality, which means we're less likely to die of *anything*.[53] There's a plethora of other health issues that exercise can either protect or help treat, ranging from chronic pain disorders like fibromyalgia, to protecting bone health and maintaining muscle mass in the elderly.[54–56] Exercise has also been shown to significantly reduce the risk of anxiety, depression and stress.[57, 58] Not only that, but for patients who already have clinical anxiety or depression, exercise has been shown to be one of the most effective prescriptions available to help treat these issues.[59, 60] Exercising outdoors when possible seems to have the greatest effect for improving wellbeing, so get outside when you can.[61]

Even in the absence of mental health disorders, exercise can boost positive feelings like happiness, enjoyment and contentment,[62] much of which is thanks to the rush of endorphins produced in response to the exercise. These endorphins, like morphine, act on the opiate receptors in our brain to reduce pain and boost feelings of pleasure. We all know the feeling sometimes known as 'runner's high', where we feel almost euphoric both during and for some time after exercise. Physical activity can energize us too – a review of 12 studies showed that exercise can have a protective effect against feelings of low energy and fatigue.[63]

Finally, from a social aspect, exercise can be a great way of bringing people together in a social environment. There's ample evidence, and even a systematic review of studies, showing the significant social health benefits of exercise, especially team-based sports.[64] Exercise has also been shown to boost sex hormones and function in both men and women, contributing to a healthy sex life, which is one of the most powerful social connections we can make and which markedly improves wellbeing.[65–68] Lastly, exercise has been shown to significantly improve sleep quality – which, as we saw in the last section, brings about many of its own health and performance benefits.[69]

Even if you are already exercising regularly, do you pay much attention to the amount of time spent sitting, or breaking up long periods of not moving? This is something I like to ask even of clients who are elite-level athletes. That's because taking part in regular exercise is all very well, but what you're doing for the rest of the day is also extremely important. Did you know that the amount of time we spend in sitting, for example at a computer, significantly influences our health, *independently* of how much we exercise? So even if you trained hard for an hour in the morning, if you spend the rest of the day sitting in your car, at a desk, then back in your car, and promptly followed by an evening on the sofa, this is an independent risk factor for many diseases that's only partially offset by the exercise. In fact, a recent meta-analysis showed a 34% higher mortality risk for adults routinely sitting more than 10 hours a day, even when adjusting for physical activity.[70] One of the mechanisms responsible for this is likely that long periods of sitting can increase markers of inflammation.[71] As we know, inflammation can affect health, but it can also disrupt the metabolism of muscle mass and so is important for athletes. So here are some easy, practical ways you could adopt to help break up long periods of sitting down:

1. Set a reminder on your phone or computer every hour to get up and walk around for a few minutes.
2. Walk or cycle at least some of the way to and from work – if you can't manage it the whole journey, you could always get off the bus a couple of stops early or park the car a little further away than usual.
3. Drink plenty of water – you'll need to get up to fill your glass or water bottle each time, as well as a few extra mini trips to the loo.
4. Design your environment for movement – move your bin, printer, and stationery away from your desk – if the bin's on the other side of the room, you'll have to get up each time you want to throw something away.
5. Chair stretches – if you can't get away from your desk, try practising a few different upper and lower

body stretches or exercises while sitting in your chair. You can find lots of free ideas for different movements online.

6. Stand up – if you're lucky enough to have a standing desk, great, use it for some time each day. If not, perhaps just try aiming to take your phone calls standing up.

7. Walk and talk – if the weather's nice, why not take a meeting outside and walk while you talk? People often find walking meetings less formal and the endorphins can help get the creative juices flowing!

8. In the evenings – stretch in front of the TV! The positions don't have to be strenuous, just getting off the sofa and relaxing in some simple yoga positions while you're watching your favourite show helps to get the circulation going.

Hopefully you can now appreciate that exercise is about so much more than just losing weight or gaining muscle. So many people focus on the outcomes and forget that movement is in fact closely related to nutrition, sleep and stress, and has profound effects on our physical, mental and social health. These effects are important even for the highest-level athlete, especially when it comes to activities outside of training, and later on when considering retirement from sport. For any readers who are less active, I'd strongly encourage you to find a sport or hobby that you genuinely enjoy, rather than working out because you feel you ought to – it's just more fun that way and you'll be much more likely to stick with it (and reap the benefits) long into the future.

STRESS

There are several definitions of stress. For most people, the word stress conjures up thoughts of mental and emotional tension or strain when we have too much on our plate. For others it could invoke thoughts of particularly demanding or uncomfortable situations. Either way, it's not a nice feeling – you might feel overwhelmed, anxious, or unable to cope as a result of pressures that are unmanageable. Of course, what contributes to stress can vary greatly from person to person and differs depending on past experiences, social and economic circumstances, the environment we live in, and even our genetic makeup. In this section, we'll consider how short-term stress can directly affect performance, as well as the effects of chronic stress on overall health and the subsequent indirect impact on your training and progress.

There are times when stress is a good thing. Let's cast our minds back 20,000 years: if our ancestors came face to face with a large sabre-toothed cat, the natural biological response to that stress would have been highly beneficial. There would have been a quick release of hormones into the bloodstream, such as cortisol, adrenaline and noradrenaline. These hormones increase energy levels and muscle tension, reduce sensitivity to pain, slow down the digestive system and cause a rise in heart rate and blood pressure. All these adaptations are designed to maximize our chance of survival against the attack so we can stay alive and pass on our genes to future generations. Those same responses, in moderation, can have performance-enhancing effects in sport too. However, too much stress, such as the anticipation of performing a pivotal sporting match or playing in front of a full stadium of fans, can result in feelings like panic or anxiety that can negatively impact performance and detract from the enjoyment of taking part. At the other end of the spectrum, too little stress can leave athletes feeling bored or unfocused, and unable to benefit from those same innate physiological responses that used to protect our ancestors. The diagram below shows how the right amount of stress can be optimal for peak performance, while both too little and too much stress can be detrimental.

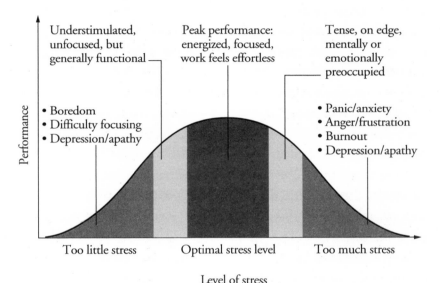

So what can we do to try and ensure our levels of stress in sport stay somewhere in that middle sweet spot?

Too little stress – this is less common but certainly affects some athletes, especially during games or races that are deemed less important or during repetitive training sessions. In these scenarios, techniques to increase a state of arousal can include mental imagery, self-talk, goal setting and focusing on thoughts that heighten stimulation.

Too much stress – sports psychologists choose from numerous different techniques to help athletes control stress before and during an event, depending on individual needs and the issue at hand. If you feel overwhelmed by stress around competitions, there are, however, a number of techniques you could try yourself, such as meditation, performance and competition planning, self-compassion, calming imagery, identifying strengths and goal setting.

What about long-term, low-level stress that we encounter in our everyday lives – can that affect performance too? Absolutely. When stress persists even at lower levels, it can affect our physical and mental health, and subsequently impact training and progress indirectly too. The type of stressors that we encounter far too often in modern society are low-grade, but frequent, or even constant. 'Microstressors' are daily hassles such as meeting deadlines for work, making difficult decisions, traffic jams or conflicts with other people. 'Ambient' stressors, as the name implies, are part of the background environment, such as noise, crowding or money worries, which can increase stress levels even without conscious awareness.

Regardless of the type of stressor, the biological response is the same, even if not quite to the extremes of an acute stressor such as imminent attack. But those responses, like raised heart rate, blood pressure, and muscle tension, aren't particularly helpful when we're late for work and stuck in a traffic jam.

Often after a single stressful situation, like playing an important sporting match in front of a crowd, we can quickly return to a resting state without any negative effects on our health. But unfortunately, many of those ambient- and microstressors are very frequent or persistent in modern society.

And if our stress response is activated repeatedly, the effects over time can result in wear and tear on the body. For example, chronic stress is linked with reduced immune system function,[72] digestive issues and irritable bowel syndrome,[73] and increased risk of stroke and heart disease.[74, 75] Stress has also been shown to significantly affect sleep duration and quality, for example a recent meta-analysis showed high stress was associated with a 73% increased risk of insomnia.[76–78] Again, this highlights just how inter-related these lifestyle factors are, and we know from the previous section how important sleep is for all aspects of health and performance. Another side-effect of chronic stress and the long-term elevation of stress hormones is higher levels of systemic inflammation,[79] which can disrupt the metabolism of muscle mass, and lead to the accumulation of fat within the muscle, both of which are undesirable for most athletes.[80]

You'll probably have felt stressed or overwhelmed at some point in time. It may have manifested in the physical consequences described above, or perhaps contributed to feelings of anxiety or depression. It may have changed the way you interact with family and friends, or even negatively affected your sex life.[81] Some people seem to be more affected by stress than others – for some, getting ready to leave the house on time every morning can be a very stressful experience. Others may be able to cope with a great deal of pressure. While it may be possible to remove or change some of the stressors in your life, others may be out of your immediate control, in which case finding mechanisms to better cope with the stressors may be more practical. Here are ten top tips for managing stress:

1. **Realize when it is causing a problem and identify the causes.** An important step in tackling

stress is to realize when it is a problem for you and make a connection between the physical and emotional signs you're experiencing and the pressures you're faced with. It's important not to ignore physical warning signs such as tense muscles, feeling over-tired, and experiencing headaches or migraines. Once you've recognized that you're experiencing stress, try to identify the underlying causes. Sort the possible reasons for your stress into those with a practical solution, those that will get better anyway given time, and those you can't do anything about. Take control by taking small steps towards the things you can improve.

2. **Review your lifestyle**. Are you taking on too much? Are there things you're doing which could be handed over to someone else? Can you do things in a more leisurely way? You may need to set yourself realistic expectations, prioritize things you're trying to achieve, and reorganize your life so that you're not trying to do everything at once.

3. **Build supportive relationships**. Finding close friends or family who can offer help and practical advice can support you in managing stress. Joining a club, enrolling on a course, or volunteering can all be good ways of expanding your social networks and encouraging you to do something different. Equally, activities like volunteering can change your perspective, and helping others can have a beneficial impact on your mood.

4. **Eat healthily**. A healthy plant-based diet will reduce the risk of diet-related diseases. There is also

a growing amount of evidence showing how a balanced vegan diet can improve emotional wellbeing.[82]

5. **Be aware of your smoking and drinking**. If possible, try to cut right down on smoking and drinking. They may seem to reduce tension, but in fact they can make problems worse. Alcohol and caffeine can increase feelings of anxiety.

6. **Exercise**. Physical exercise can be an excellent initial approach to managing the effects of stress. Walking and other physical activities can provide a natural 'mood boost' through the production of endorphins. Even a little bit of physical activity can make a difference, for example, walking for 15–20 minutes 3 times a week is a great start.

7. **Take time out**. One of the ways you can reduce stress is by taking time to relax and practising self-care, where you do positive things for yourself. Striking a balance between responsibility to others and responsibility to yourself is vital in reducing stress levels.

8. **Be mindful**. Mindfulness meditation can be practised anywhere at any time. Research has suggested it can be helpful for managing and reducing the effect of stress, anxiety and other related problems in some people, for example by reducing cortisol levels, blood pressure and heart rate.[83]

9. **Get some restful sleep**. Sleep problems are common when you're experiencing stress, but getting healthy sleep can really help with stress. Try the tips earlier in this chapter to promote good sleep habits.

10. **Don't be too hard on yourself**. Try to keep things in perspective and don't be too hard on yourself. Look for things in your life that are positive and write down things that make you feel grateful, as this has been shown to improve wellbeing.[84]*

Finally, if you feel unable to manage your stress, or have any other mental health concerns, you can find more information and support at the following sites. Some people are reluctant to seek help, as they feel that it's an admission of failure. This is not the case, and it's important to get help as soon as possible so that you can begin to feel better.

https://www.mind.org.uk/
https://www.mentalhealth.org.uk/
https://www.rethink.org/

RELATIONSHIPS

Human beings are inherently social creatures. As far back as we can trace, there's evidence that humans travelled, lived, and thrived in social groups or tribes. Those who separated from their tribe had to fend for themselves and often suffered severe consequences, facing starvation and greater threat from predators and rivals. Not only that, but social groups provided us with an important sense of identity, they taught us skills that helped us to live our lives, and they provided us with support through times of adversity. That's why

---

* Tips adapted from the Mental Health Foundation, accessed: https://www.mentalhealth.org.uk/a-to-z/s/stress.

it's ingrained in our DNA to seek and foster deep social connections.[85]

It's only in the last 250 years or so, since the dawn of the industrial revolution, that the traditional bonds of large family units and close-knit communities have changed dramatically and morphed into modern nuclear families living in separate homes, often in different cities or even countries to their extended families. We enjoy much more freedom now, from choosing where to live and what career to pursue, to how to spend our money and where to travel. But this has come at the expense of deep social connections that smartphones and computers can only partly replace. We also work long hours, which can affect the relationships even within our small households – we often don't even have much time to spend with the family we live with, and even when we do, we're often thinking about work.

I'm not suggesting you need to do anything radical like quit your job or invite your extended family to move in with you. But there are some simple and easy steps and reminders we can use to foster our relationships which can benefit your family and friends as well as yourself. Before we look at these, it's useful to know just how much our social connections (or lack of) have been shown to affect us.

Our physical health, as well as our mental and emotional wellbeing, is closely linked to our relationships. A meta-analysis reviewed 148 individual studies assessing social connections and risk of mortality, and found that people with stronger social relationships had a staggering 50% reduced risk of premature death.[86] Conversely, loneliness, which is the perceived lack of quantity and quality of relationships, has been linked with many physical diseases ranging from cardiovascular diseases, to cancer, and even susceptibility to infectious diseases.[87–89] Many people don't realize, but it seems social connections influence our health in ways that are every bit as powerful as some of the other well-established risk factors, such as diet, exercise, sleep and even smoking. Evidence of the adverse effects of loneliness on mental health is just as strong, with research showing that lonely people are at increased risk of depression, anxiety, schizophrenia, suicide, dementia and Alzheimer's disease.[90–94]

We all understand that being sociable makes us feel good. But why are social connections so impactful on our health and wellbeing? Of course, there are the practical implications of having close friends and family – they can look after us when we're ill, or provide food for us if we're unable to afford to go shopping. But the science shows there's so much more to it than that. Although there's still a lot to be discovered about the physiological responses to social interactions, research to date shows that these health benefits are likely to be largely down to complex hormonal responses that are triggered when we interact with others. For example, oxytocin is a hormone that has roles in bonding between parents and children, romantic love, friendships, and even in the bond between humans and their pets. Because its release is particularly high when we touch – holding hands, massaging, hugging and sexual intimacy have all been shown to stimulate the release of oxytocin[95] – it's sometimes referred to as the 'hugging' or 'love' hormone. But research shows that oxytocin and a related hormone called vasopressin are also released during all kinds of positive social interactions, such as meeting friends, having deep conversations, and even hearing a familiar voice on the phone.[96] These hormones feel lovely and help us navigate our world of complex social relationships by rewarding positive social behaviour with feelings of calm, closeness and love.

Many other hormones also work in concert with oxytocin and vasopressin during social interactions. For example, dopamine, a neurotransmitter involved in the reward system of the brain, creates feelings of pleasure, while serotonin, another neurotransmitter, is involved in mood regulation and contributes to feelings of wellbeing, happiness and reduced anxiety and depression.[97, 98] The reason all this is so important for improving strength and fitness is that these positive effects on wellbeing have been shown to make us more likely to maintain higher physical activity levels in the long run.[99] You're probably familiar with the scenario – sometimes heading out for training can be the last thing you want to do if you're feeling low. Healthy relationships can support wellbeing, meaning you're more likely to get out and reap all the benefits of exercise.

The other significant impact social connections can have on athletes and sportspeople is also related to hormones. There's strong evidence to show that the more socially connected people are, the less likely they are to experience chronic stress, for example with lower levels of the stress hormone cortisol.[100] This in itself brings countless physical and mental health benefits described in the stress section of this chapter, including lower levels of inflammation – which, as you now know, can significantly impact performance and training progress.

As I mentioned earlier, we don't have to do anything drastic to improve our sense of connectedness. Below are some tips that could help you to nurture and develop your social relationships. The bonus here is that as well as the potential improvements in health and performance, all these things feel lovely and help make other people happier too!

1. **Unplug**. Put your phone away when you're with friends or connecting with family. Nothing says 'I'm not listening' more than looking at your phone in the middle of a conversation. You could also try having one screen-free evening per week in your house: no TV, laptops or phones for an evening. Instead try sitting down at the table for dinner without the TV on, playing cards or board games, talking about something you're passionate about, reading to each other, giving massages, or making plans together.

2. **Embrace more.** The human touch is powerful and one of the biggest signals for the release of oxytocin, helping us to bond while feeling more contented and relaxed. When appropriate, encourage hugging, cuddling and holding hands. Giving and receiving massages has double benefits because they can help your muscles recover from exercise.

3. **Nurture your existing friendships.** Be kind. Acts of kindness have been shown to promote the wellbeing of the giver just as much as the receiver. Make yourself available. Truly listen without judgement, letting the other person know you're paying close attention with eye contact and asking further questions about their successes or problems. Show that you can be trusted and dependable, while opening up yourself, to show your friend they hold a special place in your life.

4. **Make new friends.** If you feel you could benefit from more friends, or from cultivating a more

diverse network of friends, try taking up a new interest such as a sport, a new class at the gym, volunteering locally, or dog walking (perhaps volunteering to walk dogs at your local shelter). These are all positive and active environments where you're likely to find people with similar interests. Alternatively, think back to people you've already met who made a positive impression and reach out to them, or ask a mutual friend to reintroduce you. But remember, the quality of our relationships is a far greater indicator of our wellbeing than the number of friends we have.

5. **Smile more.** Research shows that smiles really are contagious.[101] They make everyone in the room, even strangers, smile too, because humans have an instinct for facial mimicry. And smiling, even when we don't feel like it, is another trigger for the release of those hormones that make us bond and feel great – oxytocin, dopamine and serotonin. Signals of happiness like smiling have been shown to spread through three degrees of separation (e.g. to the friend of a friend's friend)![102]

After reading this chapter, I hope you can appreciate why these lifestyle factors, along with your nutrition, are so critical to your health and wellbeing. Each one is also important for performance: we've seen how healthy sleep can improve endurance performance and MPS, as well as the cognitive functions of athletes. Exercise is a key component for good mental and physical health, while breaking up longer periods of sitting can reduce markers of inflammation, resulting in the potential for improvements in muscle mass metabolism. Measures we can take to manage stress can help us reach peak performance and lower levels of chronic inflammation. And finally, nurturing strong social relationships can reduce stress and improve overall wellbeing, in turn helping us stay motivated to train.

When just one of these components takes a dip, it can affect all the others in some way. For example, if you're lonely, you might feel more stressed and less likely to exercise, which in turn could also impact your sleep and, consequently, dietary choices. This is why I felt so compelled to include this lifestyle section within this book. As you've seen, improving just one of these factors alone can have profound effects, so just imagine the power of combining the effects of all these components together, along with your plant-based nutrition! When that happens, truly magic results are seen in terms of health, happiness, and performance.

CHAPTER 9

CUSTOMIZING
A MEAL PLAN

We've covered in some depth now the components that make up a healthy plant-based diet. To many people it can all seem a bit daunting – there's lots of information to take in and you need to consider all the key micronutrients for vegans, like vitamins B_{12} and D, calcium, zinc, iodine and omega-3. On top of this, you need the right amount of energy to fuel your lifestyle and training, but not so much as to put on unwanted weight. Enough protein to promote MPS, a healthy balance of the right fats, and you need to think about getting a whole range of antioxidants and other phyto-chemicals. Or is there a simpler way to piece it all together?

While it's important to understand these components, the reality is that most of us don't have the time or inclination to think about all of them every day. A meal plan can really help to simplify all the theory we've covered into easy guidelines you can use to build on your healthy diet, to incorporate the right kind of macronutrients, all the key micronutrients, and the widest range of antioxidants and phytochemicals that you need to keep healthy and perform at your best.

The idea with building a meal plan is not to create a rigid set of rules that you have to devotedly stick to. It's just to create a framework for establishing healthy eating patterns to then set you free to eat well intuitively long into the future. Also, rather than counting calories or macronutrients precisely, we'll use daily food groups to guide our meals and snacks. This approach is much less restrictive, easier to follow, much less time-consuming, allows a wider degree of flexibility, and is a great way to promote variation in the diet.

Variation is key

We've discussed this throughout the book, but I feel the concept of adding as much variation to the diet as possible warrants another mention in this chapter too. Getting a wide variety of foods from each major food group gives us the best chance of making sure we're taking in adequate amounts of vitamins, minerals, antioxidants and other phytochemicals necessary for optimal health, performance and recovery. No single food is perfect – for example, Brazil nuts are a great source of selenium, walnuts are a good source of omega-3 fatty acids, and almonds are rich in calcium – so eating a variety of different nuts is much better than focusing on just one. Kale is a great source of calcium, but spinach is much higher in folate and magnesium. Blueberries are high in certain antioxidants, while mangoes are higher in others. By now, you'll get the idea – the more variety in the diet, the better.

That's one of the great benefits of using food group targets rather than prescribing specific foods in a fixed food plan: it guides you to apply the principles we've learnt throughout the book and input a wide variety of different foods into each group, depending on what you want to eat, and what's available, affordable, or seasonal to you. It means you can enjoy eating rather than trying to remember which foods provide which specific nutrients, because you know if you're eating a variety of foods from each group that all of the main nutrients will be covered. The table below shows some of the nutrients that are typically rich in many of the foods within each food group.

FOOD GROUP	SERVING SIZE	NUTRIENTS PROVIDED BY GROUP
Starchy carbohydrates (choose mostly whole grains and unprocessed options)	• Cooked rice, pasta, oats, quinoa and other grains: ½ **cup** • Bread: **1 slice** • Ready to eat cereal: **½ cup** • Potato: **one medium**	• All provide significant amounts of additional protein • Fibre • Great sources of a variety of vitamins and minerals such as iron, zinc, calcium, some selenium and iodine, several B vitamins and vitamin E • Wide range of phytonutrients and antioxidants
Vegetables (choose a variety of different coloured vegetables every day – make sure to include dark green, red, and orange choices)	• Raw or cooked vegetables: **1 cup** • Leafy salad greens: **2 cups** • 100% vegetable juice: **1 cup**	• Starchy vegetables provide additional carbohydrate • Fibre • All provide additional protein • Great sources of a variety of vitamins such as A, C, and K • Dark green vegetables particularly good sources of iron and several B vitamins • Brassica vegetables (e.g. pak choy, spring greens, kale) are a brilliant source of highly absorbable calcium • Wide variety of phytonutrients and antioxidants

Fruits (focus on eating a wide variety of whole fruits including berries)	· Medium-sized fruit (apple, pear, banana, orange): **1 fruit** · Raw chopped, frozen, or cooked/canned fruit: **1 cup** · Dried fruit: **½ cup** · 100% fruit juice: **1 cup**	· Carbohydrates · Fibre · Great sources of a variety of vitamins such as A and C · Wide variety of antioxidants and phytonutrients
High protein foods (focusing on variety will provide a full range of amino acids)	· Cooked beans, lentils, chickpeas: **½ cup** · Tofu or tempeh: **½ cup** · Nut or seed butter: **2 tbsp** · Nuts: **¼ cup** · Meat analogue (e.g. textured vegetable protein): **28g** · Cooked lentil or chickpea pasta: **½ cup** · Vegan protein shake or bar: **1 serving**	· All excellent protein sources · Fibre · Great sources of a variety of vitamins and minerals such as iron, zinc, calcium, selenium and B vitamins · Nuts and seeds are also healthy fat sources (including ALA omega-3 from walnuts, chia seeds, hemp seeds and flaxseeds)
Dairy alternatives	· Fortified soy, nut, oat, rice, or hemp milks: **1 cup** · Fortified soy yoghurt: **1 cup**	· Good additional sources of calcium, vitamin D, vitamin B12, and iodine (if products are fortified with these)
Oils	· Cold pressed rapeseed oil or olive oil: **1 tsp** · Fortified vegan butter: **1 tsp**	· Vitamin E · ALA omega-3 in rapeseed oil · Vitamin B12, D, and calcium (if vegan butter is fortified with these)

ENERGY BALANCE

The first step in customizing your meal plan is to estimate roughly how much energy you typically spend. This will help you get your energy balance right – where your energy intake is roughly equal to how much you're burning. Taking in too little energy relative to how much you're expending will compromise your performance and the benefits associated with training, because with limited intake, lean muscle mass as well as fat will be used by the body for fuel, which can result in reduced strength and endurance. In addition, long-term low energy intake often results in poor intake of many of the micronutrients typically found within certain food groups. Too much energy over time, on the other hand, can lead to unwanted weight gain, which could also inhibit your performance.

This doesn't mean you need to calculate your energy expenditure precisely. In fact, I would encourage you not to: it's very cumbersome and difficult – perhaps impossible – to get accurate results outside of a laboratory setting. Your daily energy expenditure will vary according to your genes, age, sex, body size, lean muscle mass, and the intensity, frequency and duration of exercise. It will also change dramatically between training phases and even with day-to-day variation in training schedules. On top of all that, the energy you spend in your non-training activities can also change significantly from day to day too. For example, you'd spend a lot more energy if you did some gardening and grocery shopping after your morning training than if you spent the rest of the day sitting at a desk.

So using a crude estimate can be a good place to start, but ongoing you should monitor your energy requirements simply by whether you feel adequately fuelled for your training and work/home life, whether you feel hungry, and whether you're losing or putting on any unwanted weight. Using these questions as cues will help you to take the guidelines from the meal plan and adapt according to your intuition.

One easy method to initially estimate your energy require-ments is to first calculate your approximate basal metabolic rate (BMR). This is the amount of energy our body uses when completely at rest, just to support vital functions like breathing, blood circulation and controlling body temperature. You can then multiply your BMR by a factor that best represents your physical activity level. This can be a really useful exercise – athletes I work with are usually surprised at how much energy they spend. For many, this revelation can be the impetus they need to eat larger meals to fuel their training, rather than restricting meals, then making up for the energy deficit by snacking on cakes, biscuits and sweets later on.

One of the most commonly used formulas to calculate your BMR is known as the Mifflin–St Jeor formula. Simply input your height, weight, and age into the corresponding formula below to estimate your BMR, expressed in calories per day:

Females	(10 x weight, kg) + (6.25 x height, cm) – (5 x age, years) – (161)
Males	(10 x weight, kg) + (6.25 x height, cm) – (5 x age, years) + (5)

Let's use an example to show you how to use the formula: a 35-year-old woman, who is 160cm tall and weighs 65kg:

$$(10 \times 65) + (6.25 \times 160) - (5 \times 35) - (161)$$

So:

$$(650) + (1000) - (175) - (161) = 1{,}314 \text{ calories per day BMR}$$

While the Mifflin–St Jeor formula is thought to be the most accurate way to estimate your BMR, it's still not perfect. For example, it doesn't take into account differences in body composition – which would affect true BMR because muscle mass has a higher metabolic rate than fat tissue, meaning it requires more energy, even at rest. Nonetheless, the formula has been shown to be the most accurate when body fat percentage isn't known, even among morbidly obese patients.[1] If you do know your body fat percentage, you could enter your details into a calculator (there are many free online versions) that uses the Katch–McArdle formula, although it should be said that most ways to measure body fat percentage have a significant margin of error, so this still won't be precise.[2]

Now you have an estimate of your BMR, you can multiply this by a factor that best describes your physical activity level (PAL) and exercise patterns, as per the table below. This will give you your approximate total daily energy expenditure (TDEE):

CATEGORY	PAL VALUE
Sedentary to light activity lifestyle Not much physical activity required for work and only occasional participation in sport or exercise. The majority of adults in the UK fall in this category.	1.4 – 1.7
Moderately active to active lifestyle Active full-time occupations, such as construction worker or waiter, or sedentary jobs but with daily performance of one hour of moderate to vigorous exercise.	1.7 – 2.0
Vigorous or vigorously active lifestyle Engage regularly in strenuous work or in strenuous leisure activities for several hours.	2.0 – 2.4
Exceptional PAL values can be as high as 5.0 – for example during 3 weeks of competitive endurance stage cycling.[3] However, levels of energy expenditure above a PAL value of 2.4 are not sustainable in the long term.	>2.4

(PAL values adapted from the Report of a Joint FAO/WHO/UNU Expert Consultation http://www.fao.org/3/a-y5686e.pdf.)

Continuing our example on page 210 of the female who has a BMR of 1,314 calories a day, let's say this person has a desk job but plays for an amateur rugby team. Between team practice and her own gym work, she trains on average for an hour a day, 6 days a week. This would put her in the 'moderately active to active lifestyle' category, so her PAL value would be between 1.7 and 2.0. So, multiplying this by her BMR would give an approximate TDEE of 2,234–2,628 calories.

CUSTOMIZING YOUR MEAL PLAN

Now that we've got a rough estimate of our energy requirements, we can use this to see how many portions of each major food group we should target on a daily basis. The following table uses data adapted from MyPlate to show you the amount of food from each major food group that's required to satisfy various energy needs. You should use this in conjunction with the food groups table on pages 207–8, which indicates what constitutes a portion of each group. Take your approximate TDEE, round it to the nearest 200 calories, and choose the corresponding number of food groups you should aim for.

This approach is not precise, and nor should it be. For example, there's a variation in the caloric content of many vegetables: 1 cup of butternut squash will contain more calories than 1 cup of cucumber. There will also be variations in the caloric content of various grains and fruits, and the various protein sources will differ a little in their protein content. So your daily caloric and macronutrient intake

CALORIES PER DAY	1,600	1,800	2,000	2,200	2,400	2,600	2,800	3,000
STARCHY CARBOHYDRATES	5 portions	6 portions	6 portions	7 portions	8 portions	9 portions	10 portions	10 portions
VEGETABLES	2 cups	2½ cups	2½ cups	3 cups	3 cups	3½ cups	3½ cups	4 cups
FRUITS	1½ cups	1½ cups	2 cups	2 cups	2 cups	2 cups	2½ cups	2½ cups
HIGH-PROTEIN FOODS	5 portions	5 portions	5½ portions	6 portions	6½ portions	6½ portions	7 portions	7 portions
DAIRY ALTERNATIVES	3 cups	3 cups	3 cups	3 cups	3 cups	3 cups	3 cups	3 cups
ADDED SUGARS (MAX)	45g	45g	50g	55g	60g	65g	70g	75g

will vary a little. One day it might be 200 calories over, and the next it could be 200 calories under. But that's fine, because your energy expenditure will change from day to day too, depending on your exercise schedule, work commitments, household chores, the amount of sleep you got, and the countless other factors that affect how much energy you spend. Nonetheless, using these food groups is a good place to start, and from there you can make adjustments if necessary.

Once you have an idea of your estimated daily portions from each major food group category, you're ready to start customizing your own plan. The easiest way to begin is to take each food group and divide the number of servings into how many meals and snacks you plan to have each day. For example, if you were aiming for 8 portions of starchy carbohydrates a day, you might decide to incorporate 2 portions with breakfast, 2 with lunch, 1 as a snack, and 3 with dinner. Repeat with the other food groups until you've divided them all throughout the day's meals. Then you can use whichever foods within those groups that you would like to eat, already have in the fridge, or choose foods that are accessible and affordable (remembering, of course, that variation is key!). If you estimated that you require over 3,000 calories a day, you may benefit from adding additional food groups to the 3,000 calorie column while also bearing in mind the tips later in this chapter for weight gain.

MyPlate recommend 3 servings of dairy (or in the case of vegans, fortified dairy alternatives) a day for everyone. You can see in the examples on pages 215 and 216–17 that this helps achieve a calcium intake well above the UK reference intake. If you can't access or don't like these, then you may need to add extra calcium-rich foods to your diet (see Chapter 5) and find alternative sources, such as supplements, for vitamins B12, D and iodine.

Here's an example of a 2,000-calorie meal plan:

MEAL	FOOD GROUP SERVINGS	SAMPLE
BREAKFAST	Starchy carbohydrates: 2 portions Fruit: 1 portion Protein: 1 portion Dairy alternative: 1 cup	1 cup cooked oats (made with 1 cup unsweetened almond milk*) ½ cup raisins ¼ cup walnuts
SNACK	Fruit: 1 portion	1 orange
LUNCH	Starchy carbohydrates: 2 portions Vegetables: 1 cup Protein: 2 portions Dairy alternative: 1 cup	2 slices wholegrain toast 1 cup tofu scramble† with 1 cup steamed broccoli 1 cup unsweetened almond milk*
SNACK	Vegetables: 1 cup Protein: ½ portion	1 cup cucumber sticks 1 Tbsp peanut butter
DINNER	Starchy carbohydrates: 2 portions Vegetables: 1 cup Protein: 2 portions	1 cup cooked long grain white rice 1 cup black beans 1 cup steamed kale Tahini dressing
SNACK	Dairy alternative: 1 cup	1 cup plain soy yoghurt**

Brand fortified with calcium, iodine, vitamins B12 and D.
**Brand fortified with calcium, vitamins B12 and D.*
† *Calcium-set tofu.*

This sample menu provides approximately: 2,055 calories, 107g protein, 413g carbohydrates, 75.8g fat, 2.7µg vitamin B12, 21mg iron, 13.4mg zinc, 1807mg calcium, 7.8µg vitamin D, 4.7g ALA omega-3 fats, 144µg iodine and 106µg selenium (calculated using the USDA nutrition database, the UK Composition of Foods Integrated Dataset (CoFID) and individual brands). This provides more than the UK reference intakes for both men and women of nearly all the key nutrients discussed in Chapter 5. Only vitamin D is slightly under the UK reference intake of 10μg/day, but remember that it's recommended everyone consider a vitamin D supplement, and it would likely be topped up by sunlight exposure during summer months anyway. This just goes to show how a balanced and varied plant-based diet can easily provide all the key nutrients you need, while supplying the macronutrients to support the growth and development of your strength and fitness.

Here's an example of a 3,000-calorie meal plan:

MEAL	FOOD GROUP SERVINGS	SAMPLE
BREAKFAST	Starchy carbohydrates: 2 portions Protein: 2 portions Fruit: 1 portion	Two slices wholegrain toast 1 cup homemade baked beans 1 cup fresh pineapple juice
SNACK	Starchy carbohydrates: 1 portion Vegetables: 1 cup Fruit: 1 portion Protein: 1 portion Dairy alternative: 1 cup	Smoothie made with: ½ cup oats, 1 cup kale, 1 banana, ½ cup mixed frozen berries, 1 serving vegan protein powder, 1 Tbsp ground flaxseed, 1 cup unsweetened oat milk*
LUNCH	Starchy carbohydrates: 2 portions Protein: 2 portions Vegetables: 2 cups	1 cup cooked quinoa 1 cup baked tempeh 1 cup red peppers 1 cup green beans
SNACK	Starchy carbohydrates: 2 portions Dairy alternative: 1 cup	1 cup muesli 1 cup unsweetened oat milk*

DINNER	Starchy carbohydrates: 3 portions Vegetables: 1 cup Protein: 2 portions	1 ½ cups cooked rice Curry containing 1 cup chickpeas, ½ cup butternut squash and ½ cup spinach
SNACK	Dairy alternative: 1 cup Fruit: ½ cup	1 cup plain soy yoghurt** ½ cup kiwi fruit

* Brand fortified with calcium, iodine, vitamins B₁₂ and D.

** Brand fortified with calcium, vitamins B₁₂ and D.

This sample menu contains approximately: 3,075 calories, 159g protein, 505g carbohydrates, 57.2g fat, 2.7µg vitamin B12, 39.1mg iron, 21.5mg zinc, 1796mg calcium, 7.8µg vitamin D, 3.3g ALA omega-3 fats, 148µg iodine and 122µg selenium† (calculated using the USDA nutrition database, the UK Composition of Foods Integrated Dataset (CoFID) and individual brand nutrition information). This example provides even more of the UK reference intakes than the 2,000 calorie example (again, with the exception of vitamin D) – which goes to show that the higher volume of food required to match the high energy output of training naturally results in increased micronutrient intake too. After a long day of training, it can be tempting to take the path of least resistance by opting for fast foods and highly processed foods, but then there's a much greater risk of not meeting the requirements for these key nutrients – as well as many others.

---

† It should be noted that the selenium content of foods varies greatly, so the actual amount may vary from the total shown here. Adding Brazil nuts to the diet (just 1–2 a day) can help significantly top up intake.

USING A DAILY CHECKLIST

Once you become familiar with customizing your meal plan, the concept should become intuitive. Rather than planning out a meal plan every day, you may find a daily checklist easier to use as a reminder. Simply tally up how many portions of each of the food groups you've had and try to match this with your daily targets:

FOOD GROUP	DAILY TARGET	TOTAL
STARCHY CARBOHYDRATES		
VEGETABLES		
FRUIT		
HIGH PROTEIN FOODS		
DAIRY ALTERNATIVES		
DAILY REMINDER TO INCLUDE: • Vitamin B$_{12}$ (from fortified foods or supplement) • Omega-3 sources (flax, chia, hemp, walnuts, plus optional algae supplement) • Selenium (1–2 Brazil nuts) • Vitamin D (some safe daily summer sunshine, fortified food, or supplement)		

ADAPTING THE MEAL PLAN TO LOSE WEIGHT

Before deciding on whether you follow advice for weight loss, you should first ask yourself why you want to lose weight. For many clients I work with, even elite athletes, it's mostly down to how they look, and in many cases, clients have tried one diet after the next for many years – they've become chronic dieters. If that sounds familiar, then I'd encourage you to start concentrating on behaviours that focus on health rather than weight. The advice throughout this book focuses on promoting a healthy, varied, balanced plant-based diet, and ensuring a wide variety of foods from each major food group will help you to eat intuitively. Ditch the strict food rules, honour your body's natural hunger and fullness signals, and learn to enjoy and celebrate your food. You may well find that some gradual weight loss is a pleasant side-effect of this mentality. But if not, that's fine too – athletes come in all shapes and sizes, and part of being a strong and successful athlete is learning to accept your body, and appreciating the amazing things it can do in sport as well as everyday life.

It might also be worth first considering whether you might have eating behaviours that could be described as disordered. These behaviours might include anxieties or fear around food, rigid food rules or restrictions, or preoccupation about food or body image for much of the day. Anyone, no matter what their age, gender or background, can develop an eating disorder, and this may be of particular interest to those following a plant-based diet, because rates of eating disorders are significantly higher among vegans and vegetarians than in the rest of the population.[4] It's important to point out, though, that veganism shouldn't be regarded as a causal factor or a trigger for eating disorders.[5] But people with a predisposition to restrictive eating may choose to go vegan because it can promote weight loss, and it's a sociably accepted way to cut out many common foods. Eating disorders are also higher among athletes, especially in sports where weight divisions apply or where you're scored for appearance.[6] So if you can identify with any of the behaviours above, it's important to know that there is lots of free help and support available, such as:

- Beat Eating Disorders: https://www. beateatingdisorders.org.uk/
- Anorexia and Bulimia Care: https://www. anorexiabulimiacare.org.uk/
- National Centre for Eating Disorders: https:// eating-disorders.org.uk/

If you're an athlete and believe that weight loss will help with your performance, the process should always begin with identifying what constitutes a realistic, healthful body weight. This should not only be based on your sports goals, but just as importantly should take into account genetic, physiological, psychological, and social factors. A healthful weight is one that can be realistically maintained, allows for improvements in your performance, minimizes the risk of injury or illness, and reduces the risk factors for chronic disease.

For many sports, a high strength-to-weight ratio is beneficial. Body weight can influence an athlete's speed, endurance, power and agility. However, too little body fat can result in the deterioration of health and performance, for example by increasing risk of osteoporosis, amenorrhoea (missed menstrual periods) and infectious diseases.[7, 8] Weight loss, by nature, means you'll be taking in less energy, which can also affect your performance. Rapid weight loss also promotes the loss of muscle mass along with fat, which can reduce speed, power and strength. This is why, if you decide losing some weight would be beneficial for your health or performance, it should always be accomplished slowly and during your off-season. During the season you should concentrate on improving your eating habits, and then embark on weight-loss efforts when you're not competing.

If after considering all the above, you decide that weight loss could be beneficial to your health and performance, you should set your goals based on the following questions:

- What is the maximum weight that you would find suitable?
- What was the last weight you maintained without constantly dieting?
- At what weight and body composition do you perform best?
- How did you derive your goal weight? Is it a healthful weight based on your own terms – not influenced by pressure of friends, family, or to prove a point?

Why 'diets' don't work

Britain is a nation of dieters – estimates show that around half of adults in the UK try to lose weight each year. But traditional weight-loss diets just don't seem to work, because around two-thirds of those trying to lose weight end up dieting all, or most, of the time.[9] Similar statistics are found in the US.[10] I'm sure you know several people, perhaps yourself, who constantly seem to be on a crash diet/weight regain cycle. That's because traditional weight-loss diets focus so much on the sole goal of weight reduction that they neglect to consider all the other complex factors that influence not only weight, but other important aspects of health and wellbeing too. They might see short-term improvements, but they simply don't work in the long run: in a meta-analysis of 29 long-term weight-loss studies, on average more than half the weight lost was regained after two years, and 80% of weight lost was regained after five years.[11] In fact, a review of 14 long-term studies showed that around half of dieters end up regaining more weight than they lost during their diets.[12] On top of this, studies show that popular weight-loss diets, including the Atkins diet, the South Beach diet, and the DASH diet, are highly likely to lead to deficiency in several micronutrients – increasing risk for many serious health conditions and diseases.[13]

A varied and balanced plant-based diet, by contrast, as we saw in Chapter 3, is supported by strong evidence to be conducive to healthy weight loss and the maintenance of healthy weight in the long term. Why can it be so effective, especially when compared to popularized weight-loss diets?

From a psychological perspective, the motives for adhering to a plant-based diet tend to be totally different from those of following a traditional weight-loss diet. The main incentive for following a weight-loss diet tends to be, somewhat obviously, weight loss. By contrast, an interesting study in Germany conducted face-to-face interviews with over 300 vegans investigating motives for their diet choices, and found that over 80% of respondents mentioned more than one motive, including animal welfare, personal health and wellbeing, and the environment, which is likely to result in long-term adherence to a plant-based dietary pattern.[14]

There are biological reasons why a plant-based diet is conducive to weight control too. Whole plant foods have a high fibre content, meaning they typically take up a larger volume than the same amount of calories consumed from meat and animal products. So eating the caloric equivalent of plant foods vs animal foods will take longer, and will take more space in your stomach, inducing feelings of fullness and satiety.

What's more, when certain soluble fibres in plant foods are included in meals, they slow down gastric emptying (the movement of food from your stomach to your small intestines) because they increase the viscosity of your stomach's contents.[15] Thanks to this effect, including them will make you feel fuller for longer, and the resulting slowed absorption of nutrients also leads to a more gradual rise in blood sugar and insulin levels after a meal.[16] Fibre from plant foods also promotes a greater diversity of healthy gut bacteria, which studies are now showing is also linked with keeping a healthy weight.[17, 18]

Your meal plan for weight loss will look very similar to an athlete looking to maintain weight, but with slightly fewer calories. This can be achieved by aiming for the number of servings from 1–2 columns to the left of your weight maintenance level in the table on page 213, which would result in a slight calorie deficit of between 200 and 400 calories less than your required energy needs. This is a level which would promote a weight loss of around a quarter to half a kilogram a week. Numerous studies show that gradual weight loss such as this is better for preserving muscle mass, strength and performance than faster rates of weight loss.[19, 20] Also, aiming for a big calorie deficit means you'd be more likely to not meet your needs for various nutrients – if you're eating less, you have less opportunity to take in vital nutrients naturally though your food.

By following the advice in this book, you'll be focusing mostly on whole plant foods, so you'll still be eating an abundance of tasty meals and may not even notice this slight calorie deficit. Healthy weight loss will be even easier when your main focus is on making healthy lifestyle choices, including good sleep habits, stress management, staying socially connected, physical activity, and making good food choices. Remember, all these aspects are inter-connected, and you'll have the greatest results, no matter what your goals are, when you develop all of these. Some other useful, proven ways to help promote gradual, healthy weight loss are given below.

Tips for promoting a healthy weight

- Focus less on the scale and more on healthful habits such as stress management, promoting good sleep, regular exercise and making good food choices. You're much more likely to maintain a healthy body weight this way rather than by following a crash diet, which as we've seen simply doesn't work in the long run and can negatively impact your health and performance.

- Spread your food intake throughout the day – 3 main meals (including breakfast) and 2 or 3 snacks works well, and prevents you becoming overly hungry at any time, which can lead to less healthy food choices.[21]
- Monitor progress by measuring changes in exercise performance, energy levels, the prevention of injuries, normal menstrual function, and general overall wellbeing.
- Evaluate your levels of exercise as well as the amount of time you spend in sedentary behaviours. Use the advice from Chapter 8 to add more movement into your days.
- Drink plenty of water – studies show it can help with both weight maintenance and those looking to lose weight.[22]
- Focus on higher fibre options – plenty of fresh fruit and vegetables over fruit juice or dried fruit, and whole grains rather than white rice/pasta/bread.
- Alcohol – if you're a regular drinker, you may find that limiting your intake of alcohol could help you achieve your weight-loss goals without making any other changes to your diet.
- Practise mindful eating – practise gratitude for your food, take away distractions such as television or phones, notice and appreciate the sensations of eating, and listen to your body for signs it is full.
- Don't look for magic – weight-loss promoting supplements, detoxes, juicing and restrictive fad diets are very rarely based on any science and can be detrimental to your health and wellbeing.

ADAPTING THE MEAL PLAN TO GAIN WEIGHT

As with weight loss, athletes looking to gain weight should do so gradually, and may be better off doing so during the off-season, because it may take time to adjust to a heavier body weight in your sport. Goals for weight gain will depend on your sport and your initial body composition – for some, increasing muscle with minimal increases in fat mass will help performance. For others, putting on muscle along with some fat can be beneficial.

When setting goals for weight gain, there are many important factors to consider:

- Your genetics: if you've always struggled to put on weight (and other members of your family may be the same), large, rapid increases in muscle mass may be unrealistic.
- Your sport: what increases in weight would be most beneficial to your performance in your given sport or activity?
- Your training programme: how often are you training? Remember that eating a caloric surplus alone will not be enough to promote muscle growth – you must also be resistance training at least several times a week.
- Your training experience: gains in muscle mass are often quickest in the first year of heavy resistance training, becoming more gradual as athletes get more accustomed to training over time.
- Your current body composition: if you're already a large athlete with lots of muscle mass, you may

need a larger caloric surplus to gain further weight. Or you may need a lower surplus if you're overweight, as some of the energy required for skeletal muscle gain can come from existing fat stores, especially in untrained individuals in the early stages of a strength training programme.

The specific amount of extra energy required will therefore vary depending on the above factors. However, a sensible starting point for most athletes requiring weight gain would be to have an additional caloric intake of around 500 calories over your maintenance energy intake.[23] This should be done in conjunction with increased strength training to provide the stimulus for MPS.[24] This could be achieved by adding an extra 2–3 portions of starchy carbohydrates and/or protein servings on top of the level you require for maintenance. However, especially for those with an already high food intake, this may be easier said than done. We've covered some tips on fuelling a highly active schedule in Chapter 7, but to recap and expand on this a little, see the list below for some advice on adopting the meal plan to promote weight gain:

- Aim for approximately 500 calories over your maintenance energy intake. If weight gain is faster or slower than you expected, adjust accordingly from here.
- This calorie surplus could be achieved through adding 2–3 extra portions of carbohydrates and proteins, and/or choosing higher-fat foods such as nuts, seeds, nut butters, avocado, and healthy dressings such as those on pages 264–8.

- Spread your food intake throughout the day rather than just going for a couple of very large meals a day to maximize MPS.
- Strength training should be a priority, to promote MPS and ensure that as much weight gained as possible is muscle mass.
- Make sure you're getting an adequate protein intake suitable for strength training athletes as detailed in Chapter 6. But bear in mind that protein intakes above this are unlikely to promote muscle growth any further.
- Choose lower-fibre foods – bulky, low-calorie foods like whole grains and salads are too filling in relation to the calories they provide. Try opting for white rice, pasta or bread options instead.
- Fruit juice, dried fruit and smoothies are all calorie-dense options that may help you increase your energy intake in addition to whole fruits.
- Make sure you're getting adequate rest and sleep between your training sessions. Remember, these are key elements to your success.
- Don't overdo it – more than 1,000 calories a day over what you need for maintenance will almost certainly lead to rapid weight gain, mostly from fat accumulation.
- Stick to healthy foods – it can be tempting to add lots of junk foods and processed foods to help bump up caloric intake – however, these foods provide little else and you may end up falling short on many micronutrients, which could hinder health and performance.

I hope after reading this chapter you understand why trying to count calories precisely is usually futile, and that using these food group targets instead can be a fantastic way to meet your nutritional needs. It's an approach that requires much less time and planning, and over time should just become intuitive, meaning long-term, sustainable results. It's also a great way to promote that all-important variation in your diet, which is critical for anyone to feel and perform their best.

The last remaining step is learning how to make delicious, quick meals and snacks to help fit in with your meal plans. Up until now we've talked about nutrition and food in a very scientific manner, but the food you eat, as well as helping support your health and athletic progress, should also be creative, artistic, and make your tastebuds dance! In the next chapter are some of my favourite recipes, as well as some guidance on how to create your own meals, so you can keep adapting with new ingredients to keep things fresh and exciting long into the future.

CHAPTER 10

THE RECIPES

A vegan diet should be one of abundance and celebration of the incredible variety of plants we can prepare and eat. While reaping all the health and performance benefits we've discussed throughout the book, we get to enjoy delicious vegan versions of cuisines from every country and culture from around the world, which to me is a win-win scenario! The food should be colourful, varied, fresh, hearty and – of course – packed with flavour.

Because you're eating predominantly whole plant foods, the diet is full of fibre, loaded with vital nutrients, and with fewer calories compared to more processed foods and animal products. So for someone who loves food and eating, like me, a real bonus to a vegan diet is getting to eat a huge amount of delicious healthy vegan meals which in turn keep me satiated and excited. Home cooking is the best way to ensure you're taking in the most important nutrients naturally through your diet. You're able to pack in the widest variety of healthy ingredients, while limiting the unnecessary excess salt, sugar and oil often found in pre-packaged ready meals and more processed foods. So I want to provide you with some delicious recipes that are really quick, easy, and efficient, to help save you time – which will hopefully in turn encourage you to cook more! These are tried and tested recipes that I cook all the time at home, and I'm sure you'll love them. There are also instructions for how to make an unlimited number of your own creations – smoothies, salads, soups, and stir-fries – so you can learn the basic principles and keep things varied, seasonal, and exciting.

I know not everyone has as much time as they'd like for cooking (me included!), so here are some quick tips I use myself to save time in the kitchen:

- Plan ahead – make a rough plan for your week's meals based on what you like, what you already have in the fridge/cupboard, and what's seasonal.

- I also recommend using the weekends to prep lots of food for the week. This can be a fun Sunday afternoon activity, and saves you loads of time during the week when you may not have as much time/energy as you'd like after work.

- Use recipes that can be made in big batches and then frozen. This way, you cook once, but have several portions in the freezer for a healthy 'instant meal' on those days when you don't have time to cook something from scratch.

- Using recipes that can be cooked and eaten as several different meals can help save time. For example, quickly roasting vegetables means they can be eaten as a snack, or used in salads,

sandwiches, pasta dishes or quick curries
throughout the week.

- Make lunch at the same time as dinner. Portion up
  salads or make sandwiches for your lunch
  tomorrow to save getting everything out again.

- Use some 'one-pot' recipes – they're easier, quicker,
  and with less washing-up at the end!

- Invest in some good-quality knives and keep them
  sharp. You'll be amazed at how much more efficient
  your meal prep will be (just watch those fingers)!

- Use tinned beans, lentils and chickpeas if you don't
  have time to cook them from scratch yourself
  (although if you do have time, the guide to cooking
  legumes and grains on page 299 will show you how
  to be more economical).

I hope using these tips will really help save you time in the
kitchen, because I'm a big advocate for making life as easy
for yourself as possible when it comes to cooking. We now
know the principles of how to optimize our healthy plant-
based diet, but if cooking were overly complicated or time-
consuming, it would make it more tempting to choose the
easy option of a takeaway or ready meal. Of course, these
kinds of foods can (and should) be enjoyed from time to
time, but they're unlikely to provide your body with as much
of the beneficial nutrition as home-cooked foods. It's the
'everyday' nutrition that counts: the kind of food you eat on
a daily basis is what will contribute the most to your intake

of key nutrients, such as those discussed in Chapter 5. The following recipes are simple and will show you how easy it is to incorporate a variety of those key nutrients regularly into your diet.

A note on measurements within these recipes: in general, I like to use cups to make life easier when it's not so important to be precise with measurements. For example, when adding ingredients to a smoothie, you certainly don't need to get out the weighing scales each time! In this instance, standard US cup measurements are used to calculate the nutrition information (which is provided **per person** in the recipes). Likewise, I usually use teaspoons and tablespoons to measure small amounts, because they're much easier. When it's a little more important to be precise in a recipe, then grams or millilitres are used.

BREAKFASTS

MY SIMPLE SMOOTHIE GUIDE

Smoothies take just a few minutes to prepare in the mornings, and they're an incredibly healthy way to start the day. They allow you to take in a huge variety of nutrients and can help you on your way to reaching the daily reference intakes for many of the nutrients mentioned in this book, before you've even left your house in the morning! Here are some general guidelines I like to follow when it comes to making smoothies:

- Get some vegetables in there – this will reduce the sugar content and increase the variety of important nutrients.
- Get a good range of colours (always including some dark leafy greens) – this will also ensure a wide variety of important nutrients.
- Top up with water or unsweetened plant milk – you need some liquid to give the smoothie a drinkable texture, but topping up with fruit juice means your smoothie will be much higher in sugar.
- I like to add 1 tablespoon of ground flaxseed, hemp or chia seeds to add some omega-3 and a little extra protein to the smoothie.
- If you're looking to top up your protein intake further, now is a good opportunity to add your favourite vegan protein shake.
- One scoop of most protein powders will add around 20g of protein.

Here's a great example:

My simple green smoothie

TIME: 5 minutes
DIFFICULTY: easy
STORAGE: best consumed within a few hours
SERVES: 1

1 banana
1 green apple
1 large handful of fresh kale
1 tablespoon ground flaxseeds
1 cup of water or plant milk

Place all the ingredients in a high-powered blender.
Blend on high until smooth.
Pour into a glass or enjoy straight out of the blender jug!

NUTRITION:

- Calories: 303
- Protein: 7.5g
- Carbohydrates: 61.0g
- Of which sugars: 36.5g
- Fats: 4.7g
- Of which saturates: 0.7g
- Fibre: 12.0g

Great source of key nutrients **calcium** and **omega-3**, plus vitamins A, C, K and potassium.

MY SMOOTHIE BOWL GUIDE

Want to turn any smoothie into a smoothie bowl? It's like having a healthy ice cream for breakfast, and they're great because eating your smoothie with a spoon slows down your eating. Plus you can appreciate the nice toppings which add different colours and texture. Just follow these steps:

- Peel, chop and freeze your bananas – the high pectin content means that when frozen and blended they help to create an incredibly smooth, 'soft serve ice cream' type texture.

- Reduce the amount of water or liquid by around half to help keep it thick.

- Blend on high until it is thick and smooth; you may have to scrape down the sides of the blender a couple of times.

- Top with anything you like! Favourites for me are fresh fruit, granola, nuts, seeds, desiccated coconut or nut butter.

Here's an example:

Blueberry protein smoothie bowl

TIME: 5 minutes
DIFFICULTY: easy
STORAGE: best consumed immediately
SERVES: 1

1 frozen chopped banana
½ cup of frozen blueberries
1 cup of fresh spinach (approx. 30g)
¼ of a fresh beetroot
1 tablespoon ground flaxseeds
1 scoop of vegan vanilla protein powder (optional)
½ cup of water

Blend all the ingredients in a high-powered blender until thick and smooth. If you like, you can then scatter over your favourite toppings, for example more fresh fruit, nuts, seeds, or nut butter.

NUTRITION:

- Calories: 294
- Protein: 27.9g
- Carbohydrates: 42.4g
- Of which sugars: 23.2g
- Fats: 4.8g
- Of which saturates: 0.5g
- Fibre: 10.2g

High in protein and a great source of key nutrients **iron** and **omega-3**, plus vitamins A, C, K, folate and magnesium.

1,000 CALORIE SMOOTHIE

Here's an example of how you can make a smoothie much more calorific to help fuel a highly active exercise schedule. We've taken some tips from Chapter 7 and have added dried fruit, nut butter and extra carbohydrate (in the form of oats and another banana) to make this smoothie much more energy-dense, as an easy way to add calories to the diet, if required. You may need a larger blender jug for this one!

TIME: 5 minutes
DIFFICULTY: easy
STORAGE: best consumed within a few hours
SERVES: 1

2 bananas
½ cup of frozen blueberries
1 apple
3 large pitted dates
1 large handful of kale
1 tablespoon flaxseeds
1 tablespoon peanut butter
½ cup of oats
1 scoop of vegan protein powder
1–2 cups of water

Place all the ingredients in a large high-powered blender and blitz until smooth.

TOP TIP:
All the smoothie examples provide a brilliant variety of fruit and vegetables. But be sure to switch things up when you can. As you know, variety is the key to success! Try kale, spinach, spring greens, lettuce or chard for your greens. Or experiment by switching the berries for some mango, the raw beetroot for some carrot, the apple for pear, etc. Sometimes adding lots of different bright colours will result in a pretty unattractive, brown smoothie, but it'll still taste great and will help you on your way to your nutrition goals!

NUTRITION:

- Calories: 1,017
- Protein: 42.4g
- Carbohydrates: 192.5g
- Of which sugars: 111.6g

- Fats: 17.1g
- Of which saturates: 2.6g
- Fibre: 28.9g

High in protein and a great source of key nutrients **calcium**, **iron** and **omega-3**, plus vitamins A, C, E, K and niacin, zinc and manganese.

OVERNIGHT OATS

If you haven't made or heard of overnight oats before, it's a method of preparing your oats without even cooking them. You simply mix them with a liquid plus any other additions, and let them rest in the fridge overnight. By the morning you'll have tender, pudding-like porridge that's extremely versatile. It takes just 2 minutes to prepare the night before, so you can have a relaxing start to the day with a bowl of nourishing goodness, with no stress or rush! You can even just grab the glass/bowl and take it to work with you.

TIME: under 5 minutes
DIFFICULTY: easy
STORAGE: 2 days in the fridge
SERVES: 1

½ cup of oats (or gluten-free oats)
½ cup of nut/oat/soy milk
2 tablespoons chia seeds
1 tablespoon agave or maple syrup

Mix all the ingredients together in a bowl, spoon into a glass or jar, and chill in the fridge overnight – simple!

NUTRITION:

- Calories: 352
- Protein: 13.3g
- Carbohydrates: 46.9g
- Of which sugars: 8.8g
- Fats: 13.4g
- Of which saturates: 1.8g
- Fibre: 15.3g

Great source of key nutrients **zinc** and **omega-3** (plus calcium, iodine, vitamin B_{12} and vitamin D if your plant milk is fortified with these).

The beautiful thing about this breakfast is that it is just as versatile as making a smoothie. Mix in whatever fruits you like, try different nut milks, leave out (or add more) sweetener, add nuts, spices, cocoa . . . the list of variations is endless, so you can get creative!

TROPICAL FRUIT:

Add ½ cup of chopped mixed fruit: pineapple, mango and banana, plus 1 tablespoon of flaked coconut.

CHOCOLATE AND PEANUT BUTTER:

Add 1 tablespoon of peanut butter and 1 tablespoon of unsweetened cocoa powder to the mix.

CARROT CAKE:

Add 1 small grated carrot, 1 tablespoon of crushed walnuts, 2 tablespoons of raisins, and ½ teaspoon of ground cinnamon to the mix.

HOMEMADE RUSTIC BAKED BEANS

This homemade alternative to tinned baked beans is much less processed and provides far more of the important nutrients, with less salt and sugar. But, just as importantly, these beans really taste way better too – delicious simply served on toast or a baked potato, or as a perfect addition to a home-cooked breakfast.

TIME: 10 minutes prep + 50 minutes cooking
DIFFICULTY: easy
STORAGE: keep in fridge for up to 3 days or freeze for up to
   3 months
SERVES: 2

1 tablespoon cold-pressed rapeseed oil
1 white onion, finely chopped
2 cloves of garlic, finely chopped
1 teaspoon smoked paprika
1 tablespoon red wine vinegar
1 tablespoon brown sugar
1 x 400g tin of butter beans, drained
200ml good-quality passata
a pinch of salt and lots of pepper
chopped fresh parsley, to garnish

Heat the oil in a large lidded pan, and fry the onion until it starts to brown, around 10 minutes. Add the garlic and paprika, and continue cooking for another minute.

Add the vinegar and sugar, then add the beans and passata. Season with salt and pepper, then turn the heat down to low and simmer gently with a lid on for 40 minutes, stirring occasionally.

Serve on toast, sprinkled with fresh parsley to garnish.

NUTRITION (1 SERVING WITH 2 SLICES OF TOAST):
- Calories: 516
- Protein: 18.4g
- Carbohydrates: 79.6g
- Of which sugars: 15.2g
- Fats: 13.0g
- Of which saturates: 1.3g
- Fibre: 11.5g

High in protein and a great source of key nutrients **iron** and **zinc**, plus copper, magnesium and manganese.

TOFU SCRAMBLE

This vegan scrambled tofu recipe is ridiculously easy – it's ready in just 15 minutes and it makes the perfect healthy addition to a vegan cooked breakfast. It's ideal for people who miss scrambled eggs, as it does look and taste somewhat similar – I'm not saying you won't know the difference, as it is tofu after all – but you may actually prefer this vegan tofu scramble!

In this version I added red pepper and shredded kale. But feel free to add whatever vegetables you have lying around – it's a great way to use them up!

TIME: 15 minutes
DIFFICULTY: easy
STORAGE: best consumed straight away, while still hot
SERVES: 2

2 tablespoons nutritional yeast flakes
½ teaspoon ground turmeric
½ teaspoon paprika
½ teaspoon Dijon mustard
½ teaspoon garlic powder
a pinch of salt and pepper
75ml plant milk
1 tablespoon cold-pressed rapeseed oil
1 red pepper, sliced
2 cups of shredded kale
280g firm tofu
optional garnish: 1 teaspoon mixed seeds and chopped fresh
coriander

First, mix the nutritional yeast, turmeric, paprika, mustard, garlic
powder, salt, pepper and plant milk in a small bowl, and set aside.

Heat the rapeseed oil in a non-stick frying pan. Add the red
pepper and fry for a few minutes, until starting to soften. Then
add the kale and stir through until starting to wilt.

Now add the tofu – just drain the excess liquid from it, but there's
no need to press the moisture out for this recipe. Break the tofu
up with your fingers straight into the pan, and continue to fry for
a few minutes until the tofu is just starting to turn golden.

Now add the sauce and stir through the tofu mixture. It'll seem a
little wet at first, but the tofu will soon absorb the liquid (along
with all the flavour) until it reaches a perfect scramble
consistency. Be careful not to overcook the tofu so it dries
out – you want to keep a soft scramble texture! Serve topped
with mixed seeds and coriander, if using.

NUTRITION:

- Calories: 320
- Protein: 23.4g
- Carbohydrates: 15.6g
- Of which sugars: 7.2g
- Fats: 18.0g
- Of which saturates: 2.0g
- Fibre: 5.2g

High in protein and a great source of key nutrients **iron**, **zinc**, **calcium** and **omega-3**, plus vitamins A, C and K, and manganese.

OIL- AND SUGAR-FREE GRANOLA

I love a bowl of crunchy granola, but looking at the ingredients list and nutrition info of the shop-bought varieties can be quite shocking, as most contain loads of added oil and sugar. Making your own is super-easy, tastes great, and is much, much healthier than the commercial brands. Not to mention it can be much more economical too! Try this granola with some soy yoghurt for breakfast, use it as a topping to add crunch to your smoothie bowls, or just eat it straight out of the jar for a quick snack any time of day.

TIME: 15 minutes prep + 40 minutes baking
DIFFICULTY: easy
STORAGE: keep in an airtight container for up to 4 weeks
SERVES: 8

80g pitted dates
2 ripe bananas (approx. 200g peeled weight)
2 cups of rolled oats (or gluten-free oats)

244

2 tablespoons tahini
1 teaspoon vanilla extract
2 teaspoons ground cinnamon
½ cup of crushed walnuts
½ cup of crushed Brazil nuts
a pinch of salt
100g soy yoghurt per serving

Preheat your oven to 150°C/130°C fan/300°F/gas 2.

If you are using very soft and sticky dates (such as good-quality Medjool dates), you don't need to soak them. If using slightly drier/harder dates, chop them and soak them in hot water for 5–10 minutes to soften them, then drain the water away.

Put the dates and bananas into a food processor and blend until smooth.

Put all the ingredients into a large mixing bowl: the oats, the date and banana mixture, the tahini, vanilla extract, cinnamon, crushed walnuts and Brazil nuts, and a pinch of salt. Mix well to combine everything.

Line two baking trays with baking parchment and tip half the mixture into each. Spread it out with a spoon or your fingers to form a thin layer.

Bake for 20 minutes, then break the granola into small chunks and spread them thinly back across the baking tray. Pop back into the oven and bake for a further 20 minutes, until the granola pieces turn golden, keeping an eye to make sure they don't burn, and shaking them around if some pieces are cooking faster than others.

Take out of the oven once they're all golden (they may still be soft at this stage but they will become nice and crunchy as they cool). Serve with yoghurt.

NUTRITION (SERVED WITH 100G SOY YOGHURT)

- Calories: 292
- Protein: 9.9g
- Carbohydrates: 32.3g
- Of which sugars: 12.5g
- Fats: 14.9g
- Of which saturates: 1.7g
- Fibre: 5.9g

Great source of key nutrients **zinc**, **omega-3**, **selenium** and **calcium**, plus vitamins B6, E, thiamine, magnesium and manganese.

SPICED ORANGE QUINOA PORRIDGE

Most people think of quinoa as a savoury food, enjoyed in salads, soups, or alongside stews. But in some parts of the world, such as Peru and Bolivia, quinoa has been eaten as a staple for millennia, and is a breakfast essential! This magical seed grain is full of protein, is naturally gluten-free, and is jam-packed with nutrients such as iron and magnesium. I love this version, flavoured with warming spices and some sweetness from the orange. Give it a try and you'll be set up perfectly to tackle your day!

TIME: 20 minutes
DIFFICULTY: easy
STORAGE: best eaten straight away, while still hot
SERVES: 1

100g quinoa

1 tablespoon chia seeds

1 teaspoon ground cinnamon

½ teaspoon ground turmeric

¼ teaspoon ground ginger

¼ teaspoon ground mixed spice

juice of 1 orange

200ml soy or other plant-based milk

1 teaspoon maple syrup

In a saucepan, mix the quinoa with the chia seeds and spices.

Add the orange juice, plant milk and maple syrup and stir to combine. Bring to the boil, then simmer for 15–20 minutes, until the quinoa is soft, tender, and has soaked up most of the liquid.

Transfer to a bowl and add your favourite toppings – fresh or dried fruit, nut butters and desiccated coconut all work well.

NUTRITION:

- Calories: 560
- Protein: 22.9g
- Carbohydrates: 85.3g
- Of which sugars: 20.0g
- Fats: 14.1g
- Of which saturates: 1.7g
- Fibre: 13.5g

High in protein and a great source of key nutrients **iron**, **omega-3** and **zinc** (plus calcium, iodine, vitamins B_{12} and D if your plant milk is fortified with these).

LUNCHES

STICKY ROASTED VEGETABLES

These are so incredibly easy, healthy and versatile. Prepping them at the weekend is super-quick, and will save you time during the week by providing you with really tasty vegetables to quickly chuck into pastas, curries, sandwiches and salads over the next few days. We roast vegetables most weeks in our house so we can whip up a fast meal when time is short.

TIME: 15 minutes prep + 40 minutes roasting
DIFFICULTY: easy
STORAGE: keep for up to 3 days in the fridge
SERVES: 4

1 aubergine, cut into bite-size chunks
1 courgette, cut into bite-size chunks
1 red onion, cut into wedges
1 red pepper, sliced into thick chunks
2 x 400g tins of chickpeas, drained and rinsed
2 tablespoons rapeseed oil
a pinch of salt and pepper
3 cloves of garlic, sliced

Preheat the oven to 180°C/160°C fan/350°F/gas 4.

In a large bowl, toss all the chopped veg and chickpeas with the rapeseed oil, salt, and pepper, then lay out on two baking trays (trying to minimize overlapping as much as possible). Roast for about 20 minutes, then remove, add the sliced garlic, toss the veg around, and pop back into the oven for another 15–20 minutes, or until the veg are all tender, browned, and nicely caramelized.

NUTRITION:

- Calories: 163
- Protein: 11.8g
- Carbohydrates: 33.4g
- Of which sugars: 6.8g
- Fats: 8.8g
- Of which saturates: 0.8g
- Fibre: 12.4g

Great source of key nutrient **iron**, plus vitamins C, K, riboflavin, potassium, manganese and folate.

LENTIL TABBOULEH

One of the easiest recipes ever, so it's a brilliant go-to dish when you're short on time! Makes a delicious light meal in itself, or you can serve it as a side with barbecued veg skewers or veggie burgers.

TIME: 30 minutes
DIFFICULTY: easy
STORAGE: keep covered in the fridge for up to 3 days
SERVES: 4

200g uncooked Puy lentils (or 2 x 250g packs of cooked
Puy lentils)
200g good-quality cherry tomatoes, halved
a bunch of spring onions, finely sliced
a large bunch of fresh parsley, chopped
a large bunch of fresh mint, chopped
4 tablespoons extra virgin olive oil
juice of 1 lemon
salt and pepper

Rinse the lentils under cold water, then cook as per the packet
instructions (or use the instructions on page 299). Once tender,
rinse with cold water to cool, then drain.

Put the cherry tomatoes, spring onions, and herbs into a bowl.
Stir in the drained lentils, olive oil and lemon juice, and season
with salt and pepper to taste.

NUTRITION:

- Calories: 339
- Protein: 15.5g
- Carbohydrates: 30.5g
- Of which sugars: 3.4g
- Fats: 16.6g
- Of which saturates: 2.4g
- Fibre: 11.8g

High in protein and a great source of key nutrients **iron** and
zinc, plus vitamins A, C, E, folate, thiamine, phosphorus and
manganese.

BAKED SWEET POTATO FALAFELS

These are by far my favourite falafels, and they're baked rather than deep-fried like in most recipes, so they're much lower in fat. Perfect stuffed into a warm pitta bread with salad, pickles and a tahini dressing (see page 265).

They involve a little bit more preparation than some other recipes, but I promise it's worth it. Adding roasted sweet potato and garlic to the mix packs in flavour and adds moisture to the falafels. And coating them in sesame seeds ensures that they're golden and nicely crispy on the outside too. If you haven't heard of gram flour, it's flour made from chickpeas, so it's high in protein but importantly has wonderful binding properties when it cooks, so it helps to hold the falafels together. It's available from most supermarkets, and you can also find it in Asian stores or online.

TIME: 10 minutes prep, 55 minutes total baking
DIFFICULTY: medium
STORAGE: keep in the fridge for up to 3 days
FREEZABLE
MAKES: 12 falafels

200g sweet potatoes, peeled and cut into chunks

4 cloves of garlic, crushed

1 tablespoon lemon juice

1 tablespoon water

1 teaspoon sumac (optional)

1 teaspoon coriander seeds

1 teaspoon cumin seeds

1 x 400g tin of chickpeas, drained

¼ teaspoon chilli powder

2 tablespoons tahini

4 tablespoons chopped fresh coriander

4 spring onions, sliced

a pinch of salt

2 tablespoons gram flour

5 tablespoons sesame seeds

Preheat the oven to 200°C/180°C fan/400°F/gas 6.

Place the sweet potatoes, garlic, lemon juice, 1 tablespoon of water and the sumac on a piece of baking parchment or foil, wrap and seal. Roast for 30 minutes, until the sweet potatoes are soft.

Meanwhile, dry-fry the coriander and cumin seeds until fragrant, then grind to a powder in a spice grinder or a pestle and mortar.

In a food processor or using a potato masher, roughly mash the roasted sweet potatoes and garlic, the chickpeas, freshly ground spices, chilli powder, tahini, fresh coriander, spring onions and salt. Taste and add more seasoning as necessary and tahini until almost smooth. When you're happy with the flavours, stir through the gram flour.

Form into little balls about the size of a ping-pong ball and roll them in sesame seeds (you can keep moistening your hands to make the rolling easier). Lay the falafels out on a tray, flatten slightly, and roast for 25 minutes until firm and golden.

NUTRITION:

- Calories: 219
- Protein: 9.5g
- Carbohydrates: 27.6g
- Of which sugars: 2.7g
- Fats: 8.1g
- Of which saturates: 1.1g
- Fibre: 7.5g

High in protein and a great source of key nutrients **iron**, **zinc** and **calcium**, plus vitamins A, B$_6$ and C, folate, potassium and manganese.

TANGY SMASHED CHICKPEA SANDWICH

I love this sandwich filling – the tang from the gherkins and vinegar with the power of the onion and mustard really packs a punch. Plus many of the ingredients are cupboard staples, so you may have most of what you need lying around already.

TIME: 10 minutes
DIFFICULTY: easy
STORAGE: keep covered in the fridge for up to 3 days
SERVES: 2

1 x 400g tin of chickpeas, drained

1 medium pickled gherkin, finely chopped

¼ of a red onion, finely chopped

2 tablespoons oat crème fraiche (or sub 1 tablespoon vegan mayo)

1 teaspoon wholegrain mustard

2 teaspoons apple cider vinegar

2 teaspoons chopped fresh dill

⅛ teaspoon ground turmeric

a pinch of salt and pepper

TO SERVE

2 slices of whole wheat bread (or gluten-free bread) per person

salad leaves

grated carrot

Lightly crush the chickpeas in a bowl, using a potato masher or just the back of a spoon. It's nice to have them mostly crushed but with some of the chickpeas left whole for texture.

Mix in all the rest of the filling ingredients, then spread half the mixture between the 2 slices of wholegrain bread and top with salad leaves or grated carrot.

NUTRITION:

- Calories: 341
- Protein: 18.5g
- Carbohydrates: 49.2g
- Of which sugars: 5.8g

- Fats: 5.5g
- Of which saturates: 1.7g
- Fibre: 12.7g

High in protein and a great source of key nutrients **iron** and **zinc**, plus vitamin B_6, folate, copper and manganese.

MY TEMPLATE FOR 1,000 SOUPS!

Use the examples opposite to make a lifetime of different soups. Be experimental, you'll soon learn which flavours go best with each other, and try other ingredients too – soup's a great way to use up any leftover vegetables you have lying around! To save time I often use tinned pulses as a source of protein, but if you prefer soaking and cooking them yourself, I've included a handy guide on page 299 for cooking pulses and grains.

BASE LAYER	ADD ALL 4 BASE LAYER INGREDIENTS			
	1 onion or leek	2 sticks celery	2 carrots	3 cloves of garlic
MAIN BODY	1 CUP PER PERSON			
	Broccoli	Cauliflower	Celeriac	Tomatoes	Butternut squash
SUPPORTING VEGETABLE	1 CUP PER PERSON			
	Asparagus	Peas	Spinach	Courgette	Kale
PROTEIN	1 CUP PER PERSON			
	Quinoa (cooked)	Tinned kidney beans	Tinned chickpeas
	Tinned black beans	Tinned lentils	
HERB / SPICE	½ CUP PER PERSON / SPICES TO TASTE			
	Soft herbs: basil, parsley, coriander, or tarragon	Woody herbs: rosemary, thyme, or oregano	Cumin, paprika, turmeric, curry spice mix	Chilli flakes or powder
FINISHING TOUCH	TO TASTE		
	Toasted seeds	Plain soy yoghurt	Toasted nuts
	More fresh herbs	Drizzle of olive oil	

1 Finely chop all the **base layer ingredients**, then fry them in 1 tablespoon of rapeseed oil over a medium heat until soft (5–10 minutes), adding the **garlic** (and the **spices** or **woody herbs** if using) just for the last 1–2 minutes.

2 Add the **main body** ingredient, approx. 1 large handful per person. Add enough hot stock to cover, and simmer for around 15–20 minutes, or until beginning to soften.

3 Add 1 cup of the **supporting vegetable** and 1 cup of **protein** per person, and continue to simmer for 5 more minutes.

4 Chop the **soft herbs** (if using) and stir in right at the end of cooking.

5 Now blitz (if you like your soup smooth), using a stick blender or food processor, and add one or more of the **finishing touches** to each bowl as you serve.

. . . Example: Spiced chickpea and cavolo soup

TIME: 10 minutes prep + 30 minutes cooking
DIFFICULTY: easy
STORAGE: keep covered in fridge for 3 days
FREEZABLE
SERVES: 2

1 tablespoon olive oil, plus extra for drizzling
1 white onion, finely diced
1 stick of celery, finely diced
1 small carrot, finely diced

3 cloves of garlic, finely chopped

1 teaspoon ground cumin

1 teaspoon chilli powder

1 tablespoon paprika

2 handfuls of chopped fresh tomatoes (3 medium-size)

750 ml vegan stock

1 x 400g tin of chickpeas, drained

2 large handfuls of fresh cavolo nero, stripped from the stalks

a small bunch of fresh coriander, chopped

2 tablespoons toasted pumpkin seeds

Heat the olive oil in a large pan. Add the onion, celery and carrot and gently fry for 5–10 minutes, until soft. Add the garlic, cumin, chilli and paprika and continue to fry for a further 1–2 minutes.

Add the chopped tomatoes and the hot stock, stir, then simmer for about 15 minutes. Now add the chickpeas and the cavolo nero and stir through for 5 minutes, until the cavolo has wilted.

Take off the heat and stir in the coriander. Serve in bowls and top with a little drizzle of olive oil and the toasted pumpkin seeds.

NUTRITION:

- Calories: 391
- Protein: 16.8g
- Carbohydrates: 45.1g
- Of which sugars: 12.3g
- Fats: 12.2g
- Of which saturates: 1.3g
- Fibre: 15.1g

High in protein and a great source of key nutrients **calcium**, **iron** and **zinc**, plus vitamins A, B₆, C, K, folate, copper, magnesium, and manganese.

257

BROAD BEAN AND MINT BRUSCHETTA

Bruschetta is often served as an antipasto (starter) dish in Italy and consists of grilled bread rubbed with garlic and topped with oil and various other ingredients. The joy of this is that you can top it with just about anything (simple tomato and fresh basil is a classic) and it makes a delicious and impressive quick lunch. Here's one of my favourite variations, topped with an easy but really tasty broad bean and mint mixture.

TIME: 15 minutes prep + 10 minutes cooking
DIFFICULTY: easy
STORAGE: keep the broad bean mash covered in the fridge for up to 3 days
SERVES: 2

250g frozen baby broad beans
juice of ½ a lemon
a handful of fresh mint, roughly chopped
2 tablespoons extra virgin olive oil
salt and pepper
4 slices of good-quality bread (or gluten-free bread)
1 clove of garlic
2 tablespoons hemp seeds
a pinch of dried chilli flakes (optional)

Tip the frozen broad beans into a bowl and cover them with boiling water from the kettle, then leave to defrost. Check that they're soft after a few minutes, then drain them. If you can't find baby broad beans, larger beans may require boiling in water for 3–4 minutes to soften, then refreshing in ice-cold water. If you want, you can also double pod the beans at this stage: just pinch them to puncture the skins, and gently squeeze the tender, bright green beans out. This step is optional, as the skins of baby broad beans are quite soft, but is recommended if using older, larger broad beans. I often double pod about half the broad beans to show off their vibrant colour, while keeping a bit of texture with some of the skins.

Now roughly mash the beans with a potato masher or the back of a fork, and stir in the lemon juice, chopped mint, 1 tablespoon of the olive oil, and salt and pepper to taste.

Heat a griddle pan until it's very hot, then toast the bread for about 2–3 minutes on each side without moving it, until it has charred griddle lines across it. Alternatively, you can just toast the bread in a toaster, but you won't have the nice char marks.

Now, without peeling the clove of garlic, cut it in half. Rub the cut edge of the garlic over both sides of the toast, then drizzle over the remaining tablespoon of oil. Top the grilled garlicky bread with the broad bean mixture, and garnish with the hemp seeds and chilli flakes.

NUTRITION (PER 2 SLICES):

- Calories: 491
- Protein: 20.6g
- Carbohydrates: 61.7g
- Of which sugars: 4.9g
- Fats: 20.7g
- Of which saturates: 1.9g
- Fibre: 12.8g

High in protein and a great source of key nutrients **iron**, **zinc**, and **omega-3**, plus vitamin C, folate, magnesium, copper and manganese.

DELI-STYLE RED LENTIL PASTA SALAD

Lentil or chickpea pasta is an ingenious swap you can make that provides tons of protein and is suitable for anyone who's gluten-free. This delicious recipe serves 2, so you can enjoy it for dinner and keep the rest in the fridge for lunch later in the week.

TIME: 10 minutes prep + 8 minutes cooking
DIFFICULTY: easy
STORAGE: keep covered in fridge for up to 3 days
SERVES: 2

150g red lentil or chickpea pasta
100g frozen peas
1 large ripe tomato
10 sun-dried tomatoes, sliced
2 tablespoons olive oil
1 tablespoon white wine vinegar
1 clove of garlic, peeled and roughly chopped
a large handful of fresh basil leaves, roughly chopped
100g drained artichoke hearts, roughly chopped

First, cook the pasta as per the packet instructions until al dente (cooked but still with a bite). Add the peas to the pasta water for the last 2 minutes of cooking, then drain the pasta and peas in a colander, cool under cold running water to keep the peas vibrant, and leave to drain while you make the dressing.

Chuck the ripe tomato, half the sun-dried tomatoes, the olive oil, vinegar and garlic into a food processor and blitz to form a dressing. In a large bowl, mix the drained pasta and peas with the tomato dressing.

Stir in the remaining sun-dried tomatoes, basil leaves and drained artichoke hearts.

NUTRITION:
- Calories: 498
- Protein: 25.5g
- Carbohydrates: 52.7g
- Of which sugars: 8.5g
- Fats: 19.6g
- Of which saturates: 2.9g
- Fibre: 13.2g

High in protein and a great source of key nutrients **iron** and **zinc**, plus vitamins C, E, K, thiamine, folate and manganese.

MY TEMPLATE FOR 1,000 SALADS!

When people think of salads, they often just think of lettuce, tomato and cucumber. But when well planned, salads can be bold, exciting, colourful, hearty and of course delicious!

When I start making a salad, I like to try and make sure it has the following elements:

- Different textures – adding textures is a quick way to improve ANY dish.

- Lots of colours – makes it more visually pleasing and helps to ensure a variety of nutrients.

- Some protein – makes it more hearty and filling.

- Lots of herbs – for adding fresh bold flavour.

- Tanginess – usually from a dressing, to make your tastebuds dance!

- Some fat – also usually from a dressing, to help fuse all the above elements together.

	2 CUPS (SHREDDED) PER PERSON		
LEAVES	Fresh spinach	Blanched kale	Rocket
	Watercress	Lettuce	Blanched spring greens
DELICIOUS VEGETABLES	1 CUP PER PERSON		
	Blanched peas	Sweetcorn	Roasted peppers
	Fresh tomatoes, chopped	Roasted broccoli	Blanched green beans
TEXTURE	2 TBSP PER PERSON		
	Toasted seeds	Pomegranate seeds	Radishes, chopped
	Raw fennel, sliced	Toasted nuts	Wholegrain croutons
HERBINESS	½ CUP PER PERSON		
	Basil	Coriander	Mint
	Parsley	Tarragon	Dill
PROTEIN	½ CUP PER PERSON		
	Lentils	Quinoa	Chickpeas
	Butter beans	Kidney beans	Tofu
DRESSING	2 TBSP PER PERSON		
	Tahini (page 265)	Avocado (page 266)	Peanut satay (page 265)
	Ginger and miso (page 267)	Olive oil and lemon juice	

When you get all these elements in one salad, you create something truly magical. And once you get used to this way of building a salad, the combinations are limitless! It's a great way to get loads of variation on one plate, and these kinds of salads make a perfect lunch, dinner or side dish to sharing foods like barbecues or picnics.

. . . Example: Lettuce, pea and lentil salad with basil, toasted cashews and tahini dressing

TIME: 10 minutes
DIFFICULTY: easy
STORAGE: keep covered in the fridge for up to 3 days
SERVES 2 AS A MAIN

1 cup of frozen green peas
4 tablespoons of cashews
4 cups of Cos lettuce
1 cup of fresh chopped tomatoes
1 cup of fresh basil
1 cup of cooked Puy (or brown) lentils
4 tablespoons tahini dressing (see page 264)

To blanch your peas, put them into a small pan of boiling water, bring the water back to the boil and simmer for 1 minute. Drain the peas in a sieve under cold water to keep them fresh and vibrant in colour.

To toast the cashews, simply place them in a frying pan without any oil over a medium-high heat. Keep shaking the pan so they don't burn and toast them for around 3–4 minutes, until they're just starting to colour and smell fragrant. Alternatively you can put them on a baking tray and roast for 6–7 minutes at 180°C/160°C fan/350°F/gas 4.

Put all the ingredients into a large bowl and mix to combine.

NUTRITION:

- Calories: 428
- Protein: 22.5g
- Carbohydrates: 46.8g
- Of which sugars: 11.8g
- Fats: 18.0g
- Of which saturates: 2.8g
- Fibre: 15.2g

High in protein and a great source of key nutrients **iron**, **zinc** and **calcium**, plus vitamins A, C, K, thiamine, folate, magnesium and manganese.

FOUR OIL-FREE DRESSINGS

I don't mind using a little oil in my cooking, because it helps so much with the cooking process and can make food taste really delicious. But when making dressings, I often like to use whole foods as a healthy source of fat instead, such as tahini, avocado, and nut or seed butters. This means they still provide the fat that helps to bring all the elements of the dish together, but they also bring lots of other nutrients, like protein, fibre, and many other vitamins and minerals which wouldn't be found in oil.

These dressings are great on salads, of course, but can be used on loads of other dishes – they can turn a humble bowl of rice, veg and beans into a really delicious meal!

Simple tahini dressing

TIME: 5 minutes
DIFFICULTY: easy
STORAGE: keep covered in the fridge for up to a week
MAKES: 8 tablespoons of dressing

4 tablespoons light tahini
2 teaspoons maple syrup
1 tablespoon fresh lemon juice
1 tablespoon soy sauce (or 1 teaspoon tamari for GF option)
2–3 tablespoons water

Blend everything together in a cup, using a fork, or in a small blender/food processor. Taste and adjust the flavours – more lemon for tanginess, maple syrup for sweetness, soy sauce for saltiness and more water to make it thinner if needed.

NUTRITION (PER 2 TABLESPOONS OF DRESSING):

- Calories: 103
- Protein: 2.9g
- Carbohydrates: 6.9g
- Of which sugars: 3.2g
- Fats: 8.1g
- Of which saturates: 1.1g
- Fibre: 1.4g

Peanut satay dressing

TIME: 5 minutes
DIFFICULTY: easy
STORAGE: keep covered in the fridge for up to a week
MAKES: 12 tablespoons of dressing

a thumb-size piece of fresh ginger
6 tablespoons peanut butter
1 tablespoon soy sauce (or 1 teaspoon tamari for GF option)
2 teaspoons rice wine vinegar
2 teaspoons maple syrup
juice of 1 lime
1 small clove of garlic, finely chopped
1 red chilli, finely chopped
4–6 tablespoons water

Grate the ginger, then squeeze it in your hand to extract the juice into a small bowl. Discard the pulp.

Add all the other ingredients, and blend everything together using a fork. Taste and adjust the flavours – more lime or vinegar for tanginess, maple syrup for sweetness, soy sauce for saltiness, chilli for heat, and more water to make it thinner if needed.

NUTRITION (PER 2 TABLESPOONS OF DRESSING):

- Calories: 94
- Protein: 3.9g
- Carbohydrates: 3.5g
- Of which sugars: 1.4g
- Fats: 8.0g
- Of which saturates: 1.3g
- Fibre: 1.3g

Avocado dressing

TIME: 5 minutes
DIFFICULTY: easy
STORAGE: keep covered in the fridge for up to 3 days
MAKES: 1½ cups of dressing

1 medium avocado

juice of 1 lime

1 date

a handful of fresh coriander

1 clove of garlic, finely chopped

1 spring onion

1 red chilli (optional)

1 cup of water

salt and pepper

Put all the ingredients into a blender and blitz until smooth. Taste and adjust the flavours – in this one we have lime juice for tanginess, date for sweetness, coriander for herbiness and salt for saltiness.

NUTRITION (PER 2 TABLESPOONS OF DRESSING):

- Calories: 69
- Protein: 1.0g
- Carbohydrates: 6.9g
- Of which sugars: 3.1g
- Fats: 4.9g
- Of which saturates: 0.7g
- Fibre: 2.8g

Ginger and miso dressing

TIME: 5 minutes

DIFFICULTY: easy

STORAGE: keep covered in the fridge for up to 3 days

MAKES: 10 tablespoons of dressing

a thumb-size piece of fresh ginger

1 tablespoon white or brown miso paste

2 tablespoons tahini

4 tablespoons rice wine vinegar
1 tablespoon agave or maple syrup
1 clove of garlic, finely chopped
1 tablespoon soy sauce

Grate the ginger, then squeeze it in your hand to extract the juice into a small bowl. Discard the pulp.

Add all the other ingredients, and blend everything together using a fork. Taste and adjust the flavours – more vinegar for tanginess, maple/agave syrup for sweetness, soy sauce for saltiness, garlic or ginger for zing, and a dash of water to make it thinner if needed.

NUTRITION (PER 2 TABLESPOONS OF DRESSING):

- Calories: 57
- Protein: 1.6g
- Carbohydrates: 5.4g
- Of which sugars: 2.7g
- Fats: 3.4g
- Of which saturates: 0.5g
- Fibre: 0.8g

DINNERS

EASY VEGAN BURGERS

Having tried dozens of vegan burger recipes, this one hits that magical sweet spot of being easy, but tasting really great. Serve in a bun with avocado, tomato and red onion, and a drizzle of sweet chilli sauce if you like. Before cooking, the burgers can also be frozen – simply defrost them in the fridge for at least a few hours, then cook as below.

TIME: 15 minutes prep + 10 minutes cooking
DIFFICULTY: easy
STORAGE: keep burgers covered in fridge for up to 3 days
FREEZABLE
MAKES: 4 burgers

3 tablespoons cold-pressed rapeseed oil
1 white onion, finely diced
3 cloves of garlic, finely chopped
2 x 400g tins of chickpeas, drained
a handful of fresh coriander
1 teaspoon paprika
1 teaspoon ground cumin
1 teaspoon ground coriander seeds
4 tablespoons plain flour (or GF flour)
a pinch of salt and pepper

First, fry your onion – heat 1 tablespoon of the rapeseed oil in a frying pan over a medium heat, then add the onion and stir occasionally for around 10 minutes, until softening and turning translucent. Add the garlic and continue to fry for another 1–2 minutes, then take off the heat and set aside.

Drain the chickpeas well and put them into a food processor along with the cooked onion and garlic, the fresh coriander leaves, the paprika, cumin, ground coriander seeds, flour, salt and pepper. Blitz until a thick burger mixture has formed (you may need to scrape the sides of the food processor down a couple of times during the blitzing).

Shape the mixture into 4 burger patties. Heat the remaining 2 tablespoons of rapeseed oil in a non-stick frying pan, then fry the burgers on each side for 4–5 minutes or until they have nice golden, crispy sides.

Serve each burger in a bun with ¼ of an avocado, ½ a sliced tomato, a few slices of red onion, 1 tablespoon of vegan mayo and 1 tablespoon of sweet chilli sauce. This goes brilliantly with regular or sweet potato wedges.

NUTRITION (PER BURGER SERVED IN A BUN, WITH SUGGESTED TOPPINGS: ¼ OF AN AVOCADO, ½ A TOMATO, ¼ OF A RED ONION AND 1 TABLESPOON OF SWEET CHILLI SAUCE):

- Calories: 622
- Protein: 18.5g
- Carbohydrates: 77.9g
- Of which sugars: 16.1g
- Fats: 24.7g
- Of which saturates: 2.9g
- Fibre: 17.2g

High in protein and a great source of key nutrients **iron** and **zinc**, plus vitamin B$_6$, folate, phosphorus and manganese.

TERIYAKI BAKED TOFU WITH PAK CHOY

This is real comfort food – it's got all the delicious sweet, salty and aromatic flavours and is high in protein. Serve on its own for a light dinner, or with rice to make it more substantial.

TIME: 10 minutes prep + 30 minutes cooking
DIFFICULTY: medium
STORAGE: best eaten straight away while hot but can be kept in the fridge for up to 3 days and reheated
SERVES: 2

400g tofu
3 teaspoons cornflour
4 tablespoons soy sauce (or 2 tablespoons tamari for GF)
1 tablespoon rapeseed oil
1 tablespoon rice wine vinegar
1 tablespoon brown sugar
1 teaspoon toasted sesame oil
1 teaspoon fresh ginger, finely chopped or grated
1 clove of garlic, finely chopped
2 whole pak choy
1 teaspoon sesame seeds
2 spring onions, finely chopped

Preheat your oven to 180°C/160°C fan/350°F/gas 4. Carefully squeeze the tofu to get rid of excess moisture, then cut it into bite-size pieces.

In a small bowl, mix 1 teaspoon of cornflour, 2 tablespoons of soy sauce, the rapeseed oil, and toss the tofu through the marinade gently until it is all coated. Spread the tofu pieces on a baking tray lined with baking paper, and bake for 25–30 minutes, flipping the pieces halfway through, until golden and crispy.

Meanwhile, make the teriyaki sauce by combining the remaining 2 tablespoons of soy sauce, the remaining 2 teaspoons of cornflour, the rice wine vinegar, sugar, sesame oil, ginger, garlic and around 100ml of water. Mix together and bring to a simmer in a small pan. Stir occasionally until the sauce thickens (about 3–4 minutes), adding a little more water if it becomes too thick.

Separate the pak choy leaves and blanch them in boiling water for just 3–4 minutes. Drain, then lay the pak choy leaves on a plate and top with the crispy tofu and the teriyaki sauce, and scatter over the sesame seeds and chopped spring onions.

NUTRITION:

- Calories: 435
- Protein: 30.4g
- Carbohydrates: 24.3g
- Of which sugars: 10.8g
- Fats: 25.3g
- Of which saturates: 3.1g
- Fibre: 4.6g

High in protein and a great source of key nutrients **iron**, **zinc** and **calcium**, plus vitamin A, potassium, copper and manganese.

BUTTER BEAN AND VEGAN SAUSAGE STEW

This is a great recipe for using up leftover vegan sausages. I generally stick to whole plant foods and minimize processed foods like vegan sausages, but they can certainly be a part of a healthy diet when included from time to time. If I'm having them as part of a cooked breakfast, I like to cook an extra pack so I have some leftovers to make this sausage and butter bean stew – it's a really hearty and warming dish that goes brilliantly with mashed potato or even just with crusty bread.

TIME: 10 minutes prep + 60 minutes cooking
DIFFICULTY: easy
STORAGE: keep covered in the fridge for up to 3 days
FREEZABLE
SERVES: 4

1 tablespoon rapeseed oil
1 white onion, finely chopped
3 cloves of garlic, finely chopped
1 medium carrot, chopped into small pieces
1 medium parsnip, chopped into small pieces
100ml red wine
2 x 400g tins of chopped tomatoes
2 tablespoons tomato purée
1 tablespoon balsamic vinegar
1 tablespoon soy sauce
250ml veg stock
1 x 400g tin of butter beans, drained
4 cooked vegan sausages (I use soy-based varieties because
    they hold together well)

1 tablespoon fresh thyme leaves, or 1 teaspoon dried thyme
salt and pepper
crusty bread and chopped fresh parsley, to serve

Heat the rapeseed oil in a large pan over a medium heat and
gently fry the onion for 10 minutes until soft and translucent.

Add the garlic and continue stirring for another 1–2 minutes.
Add the carrots and parsnips and fry for a further 5 minutes.

Add the red wine and simmer gently until the volume of liquid
has reduced by roughly half (around 5 minutes).

Add the tinned tomatoes, tomato purée, balsamic vinegar, soy
sauce, veg stock, butter beans, thyme, salt and pepper, and
simmer for about 30 minutes. Add the cooked sausages (cut into
2cm chunks), and continue simmering for another 15–20 minutes,
until the vegetables are tender and the stew is rich and thick. Serve
hot, with crusty bread or mashed potatoes, greens (such as green
beans or broccoli), and garnish generously with chopped parsley.

NUTRITION:

- Calories: 317
- Protein: 19.2g
- Carbohydrates: 34.4g
- Of which sugars: 4.9g
- Fats: 6.6g
- Of which saturates: 0.6g
- Fibre: 12.7g

High in protein and a great source of key nutrients **iron** and
zinc, plus vitamins A and C, folate, thiamine, riboflavin,
magnesium, potassium and manganese.

MEDITERRANEAN PESTO TART

This tart is seriously simple to make, and is a delicious and healthy way to use up leftover roasted vegetables (see page 248). The pesto only takes 5 minutes to whiz up, and will leave you with about half left over, which will keep for up to a week in the fridge and can be used to stir through pasta as a post-soup topping, in salads, or as a condiment for a burger. You can even use ready-rolled puff pastry to make life easier if your supermarket sells it. Serve with a simple salad for an impressive but deceptively easy dinner.

TIME: 15 minutes prep + 25 minutes cooking
DIFFICULTY: medium
STORAGE: best eaten straight away but can be stored in the fridge for up to 3 days
SERVES: 4

1 sheet of puff pastry (320g) (or GF puff pastry)
approx. 150g fresh basil
100g walnuts
2 cloves of garlic
2 tablespoons lemon juice
2 tablespoons nutritional yeast flakes (optional)
4 tablespoons extra virgin olive oil
salt and pepper
1 cup of roasted veg (½ the recipe from page 248)
1 tablespoon soya milk

Preheat the oven to 200°C/180°C/400°F/gas 6. Use a rolling pin to roll the puff pastry sheet to the size of a large flat baking tray. Transfer the pastry to the baking tray and fold 1cm of each edge back into itself to create a double-thick border all round. Chill in the fridge while you prepare the filling.

Next make the pesto by whizzing up the basil, walnuts, garlic, lemon juice, nutritional yeast (if using), olive oil, salt and pepper in a food processor. Add a few tablespoons of water to get the right consistency – just thick enough to spread.

Spread 4–5 tablespoons of the pesto over the puff pastry, up to the border, top with your roasted veg, and brush the soy milk on to the border to help it turn nice and golden. Bake for around 20–25 minutes, or until the pastry is golden brown, then cut into 4 slices and serve with salad or roast potatoes.

NUTRITION:

- Calories: 488
- Protein: 15.4g
- Carbohydrates: 45.8g
- Of which sugars: 4.0g
- Fats: 29.4g
- Of which saturates: 10.6g
- Fibre: 8.0g

High in protein and a great source of key nutrients **omega-3**, **iron**, **zinc** (plus vitamin B_{12} if your nutritional yeast flakes are fortified).

MEAT-FREE CHILLI

I've been experimenting with vegan chillies for years now – making loads of little tweaks and improvements each time, taking inspiration from several other recipes – and I'm proud to say this is definitely the best one yet . . . It's a rich, deep chilli with a good spicy kick and complex flavours that rivals any meat-based version. The quantities in this recipe make 8 servings, so use your biggest pan and freeze any leftovers – as with many dishes, the flavours actually develop and become even more infused after freezing and reheating.

TIME: 15 minutes prep + 60 minutes cooking
DIFFICULTY: easy
STORAGE: keep covered in the fridge for up to 3 days
FREEZABLE
SERVES: 8

2 tablespoons rapeseed oil
1 large onion, finely chopped
2 red peppers, chopped
5 cloves of garlic, finely chopped
a thumb-size piece of ginger, finely chopped or grated
1 red chilli, finely chopped
1 teaspoon chilli powder
1 tablespoon ground cumin
2 tablespoons smoked paprika
150ml red wine
3 x 400g tins of chopped tomatoes
2 x 400g tins of green or brown lentils
200g quinoa, uncooked
1 x 400g tin of black beans
1 tablespoon cocoa powder
2 tablespoons soy sauce (or 1 tablespoon tamari for GF option)
1 litre veg stock
salt and lots of black pepper

TO SERVE (PER PERSON):
1 cup of cooked rice
2 tablespoons soy yoghurt
½ an avocado, roughly mashed
a handful of fresh coriander, chopped

Heat the rapeseed oil in a large pan over a medium heat. Fry the onion and red peppers for 10 minutes, until starting to soften and turning translucent. Add the garlic, ginger and red chilli and continue frying for a further 2–3 minutes, then add the spices and fry for a further 1–2 minutes, stirring continuously.

Add the red wine and let it simmer for 5 minutes, until reduced by about half. Then add all the remaining ingredients, just starting with 1 litre of stock and keeping the rest handy in case the chilli starts to look a little dry. Simmer gently for around 40 minutes, until the lentils and quinoa are tender and the chilli is deep and flavoursome.

To improve the consistency, I like to remove just a couple of ladles of the chilli and blitz in a blender to a thick sauce, then return it back to the pot (this step is optional but does give the chilli a thicker, richer consistency).

Serve with rice, and a selection of toppings such as soy yoghurt, mashed avocado and fresh coriander, sliced spring onions and pickled jalapeños.

NUTRITION (SERVED WITH 1 CUP OF WHITE RICE, ½ AN AVOCADO + 2 TABLESPOONS PLAIN SOY YOGHURT):
- Calories: 564
- Protein: 18.7g
- Carbohydrates: 86.2g
- Of which sugars: 9.8g
- Fats: 20.1g
- Of which saturates: 3.1g
- Fibre: 19.1g

High in protein and a great source of key nutrients **iron** and **zinc**, plus vitamin C, folate, pantothenic acid, magnesium and manganese.

MY TEMPLATE FOR 1,000 STIR-FRIES!

Stir-fries are always a quick, easy option in our house: once you've chopped the vegetables and got the ingredients to hand, they're ready in no time. You can make them really colourful, they're packed with protein, and with all the aromatics plus the dressing and garnishes they're always bold and flavoursome. By following these simple guidelines, your stir-fries will always have the elements of a great meal: different colours and textures, hearty protein, aromatic flavours, tanginess, saltiness and a little sweetness.

	2 CUPS PER PERSON		
2 X MAIN VEG	Red or white onion (sliced)	Broccoli (finely chopped)	Pak choy (roughly chopped)
	Sugar snaps or mangetout		Spring greens
1 X BACK-UP VEG	1 HANDFUL PER PERSON		
	Bean sprouts	Green peas	Mushrooms (sliced)
	Shredded carrots		Peppers (sliced)
PROTEIN	1 CUP PER PERSON		
	Tempeh	Tofu	Seitan
	Tinned chickpeas		Tinned black beans
AROMATICS	USE ALL 4 AROMATICS		
	2 cloves of garlic		Thumb-size piece ginger
	1 small chilli		3 spring onions

	1 CUP PER PERSON		
CARBOHYDRATE	Cooked rice	Rice noodles	Whole grain noodles
	Cooked quinoa		Soba noodles
DRESSING	USE ALL DRESSING INGREDIENTS (AMOUNT PER PERSON)		
	½ Tbsp toasted sesame oil	1 Tbsp soy sauce	1 Tbsp maple syrup or brown sugar
	1 Tbsp rice wine vinegar or lime juice		2 Tbsp Fresh coriander or basil
CRUNCH/ GARNISH	CHOOSE 1-2 TOPPINGS		
	Sesame seeds	Toasted cashews	Toasted peanuts
	Nori seaweed flakes		More spring onions

1. Prep all your ingredients in advance – stir-fries should be cooked in a sizzling hot pan, so you won't have time to be chopping veggies as you go along.

2. If using tofu or tempeh, also prepare this first – see page 292 for a great baked tofu or tempeh recipe. If adding a carbohydrate, prepare these in advance too, as per the packet instructions.

3. Heat a wok/large frying pan on a high heat, then add 1 tablespoon of rapeseed oil. Add your main veg and stir/toss in the wok for 3–4 minutes. Add the back-up veg and continue to stir-fry for another 1–2 minutes – the pan should still be sizzling hot.

4. Add the finely chopped garlic, ginger, chilli and spring onions for 1–2 minutes, until smelling aromatic.

5 Add the protein (either pre-cooked tofu/tempeh, or drained chickpeas/black beans) and the carbohydrate, and stir through for a further 1 minute.

6 Stir in the toasted sesame oil, soy sauce, maple syrup/sugar, rice wine vinegar/lime juice, and coriander/basil.

7 Serve on warm plates and choose 1–2 'garnish' ingredients to top the dish.

TOP TIP:
Keep a small cup of water nearby – if the garlic, ginger or any veggies start to burn or stick, add a small splash of water to the pan to create some steam (but not so much that you start boiling the ingredients!).

. . . Example: Tofu, broccoli and rice stir-fry

TIME: 15 minutes prep + 10 minutes cooking
DIFFICULTY: easy
STORAGE: best eaten fresh while still hot
SERVES: 2

1 serving (140g) of sriracha-baked tofu (page 292)
2 cups of cooked rice
1 head of broccoli, chopped into small florets
1 red pepper, sliced
4 cloves of garlic, finely chopped
2 thumb-size pieces of ginger, finely chopped or grated
1–2 red chillies (to taste), finely chopped
6 spring onions, finely chopped
2 tablespoons cold-pressed rapeseed oil

2 cups of shredded spring greens

1 tablespoon toasted sesame oil

2 tablespoons soy sauce (or 1 tablespoon tamari for GF option)

2 tablespoons maple syrup

2 tablespoons lime juice

4 tablespoons chopped fresh coriander

2 tablespoons toasted peanuts

2 tablespoons nori seaweed flakes (optional)

Bake your tofu as per the instructions on page 292, prepare your rice if necessary (tip: cold leftover cooked rice or packet rice works much better for stir-fries than freshly cooked) and chop the broccoli into small florets (larger pieces will take too long to cook through). Prep the rest of the vegetables. Get the rest of the ingredients ready and have a small cup of water handy in case anything begins to stick to the pan.

Heat a wok / large frying pan over a high heat. Add the rapeseed oil, then add the broccoli florets and spring greens. Stir for 3–4 minutes, then add the sliced red pepper and continue to stir-fry for a couple of minutes. The pan should still be sizzling hot.

Add the finely chopped garlic, ginger, chillies and spring onions and stir-fry for another 1–2 minutes, stirring constantly and adding a dash of water if anything begins to stick to the pan.

Add the tofu and the cooked rice and stir through to make sure everything is combined and thoroughly heated through for a couple of minutes.

Finally, stir in the toasted sesame oil, soy sauce, maple syrup, lime juice and fresh coriander.

Serve on warm plates and top with toasted peanuts and nori seaweed flakes to garnish.

NUTRITION:

- Calories: 753
- Protein: 24.5g
- Carbohydrates: 102.4g
- Of which sugars: 27.1g
- Fats: 28.9g
- Of which saturates: 3.6g
- Fibre: 13.8g

High in protein and a great source of key nutrients **iron**, **zinc**, **calcium** and **iodine**, plus vitamins C and K, phosphorus, copper and manganese.

SQUASH AND BLACK BEAN BURRITOS

Burritos are one of my favourite things to eat – mainly because they're so easy and so incredibly versatile. And you can just pack them with all your favourite ingredients! This version includes an amazing squash and black bean filling, which makes enough to fill 8 burritos. You can either freeze any leftover filling, or keep it in the fridge and enjoy it in a jacket potato or simply with some warm bread for lunch for the next couple of days!

TIME: 10 minutes prep + 60 minutes cooking
DIFFICULTY: easy
STORAGE: keep filling covered in fridge for up to 3 days
FREEZABLE (FILLING)
MAKES: 8 burritos

FOR THE FILLING (SERVES 8)

2 tablespoons rapeseed oil

1 large onion, finely chopped

4 cloves of garlic, finely chopped

4 tablespoons chipotle paste

2 x 400g tins of chopped tomatoes

200ml vegan stock

1 small butternut squash (approx. 1 kg unprepped weight), peeled, deseeded and cut into small cubes

1 x 400g tin of black beans, drained

TO SERVE (PER PERSON)

1 tortilla wrap (or GF corn tortilla)

a handful of fresh spinach leaves

¼ a cup of cooked rice

½ a small avocado, mashed with a fork

a handful of fresh coriander leaves

2 tablespoons plain soy yoghurt

1–2 teaspoons hot sauce

other optional extras: salsa, spring onions, vegan cheese, pickled jalapeños

Heat the rapeseed oil in a large pan over a medium heat. Fry the onion gently for about 10 minutes until soft and translucent. Then add the garlic and chipotle paste and continue to stir for a further 2 minutes.

Add the tinned tomatoes, stock, butternut squash and black beans, mixing everything and bringing to a simmer. Put a lid on the pan and allow to cook slowly for around 50 minutes, until the squash is tender. During this time, stir everything every 10 minutes or so to make sure it doesn't stick to the pan.

Once ready, to make one burrito, heat your tortilla wrap as per the instructions on the packet. Lay the fresh spinach leaves on the tortilla and spoon some of the squash and black bean mixture along the middle. Add the cooked rice, avocado, coriander, yoghurt and hot sauce. Be careful not to over-fill your burrito or it can be difficult to wrap up!

Fold the bottom of your wrap up over the filling. Then tuck in the sides before folding down the top edge to help keep the filling from falling out. Make more burritos the same way.

NUTRITION (PER BURRITO):

- Calories: 602
- Protein: 17.1g
- Carbohydrates: 93.3g
- Of which sugars: 9.4g
- Fats: 18.5g
- Of which saturates: 3.4g
- Fibre: 16.3g

High in protein and a great source of key nutrients **iron** and **zinc**, plus vitamins A and C, folate, thiamine, magnesium, potassium and manganese.

CHICKPEA AND SPINACH CURRY (CHANA SAAG)

Indian food has got to be one of my favourite cuisines. The flavours lend themselves so well to vegan cooking, as they're so bold and warming. This chickpea curry is super-simple but is incredibly tasty – enjoy it on its own with rice, chapattis, alongside another curry or in a jacket potato, even if it's not a very traditionally Indian thing to do!

285

TIME: 10 minutes prep + 40 minutes cooking
DIFFICULTY: easy
STORAGE: keep covered in fridge for up to 3 days
FREEZABLE
SERVES: 4

2 tablespoons rapeseed oil
2 large onions, diced
2 teaspoons cumin seeds
1 teaspoon brown mustard seeds
5 cloves of garlic, finely chopped
a thumb-size piece of ginger, finely chopped
1 teaspoon chilli powder
1 tablespoon ground coriander
1 teaspoon ground turmeric
2 x 400g tins of chopped tomatoes
200ml vegan stock
2 x 400g tins of chickpeas, drained
salt and pepper
500g baby spinach

Heat the rapeseed oil in a large pan over a medium heat and fry
the onion gently for about 5 minutes, until beginning to soften.
Add the cumin seeds and brown mustard seeds along with the
garlic and ginger. Stir constantly for about 1 minute, or until the
mustard seeds begin to pop.

Now add the chilli powder, ground coriander and ground
turmeric and continue to stir constantly for another minute,
until all the spices become fragrant. If the spices begin to stick,
add a small splash of water. Add the tinned tomatoes, stock and

chickpeas, season with salt and pepper, mix thoroughly and simmer for around 30 minutes, until the curry is thick and rich.

Add the spinach at the end, pushing it into the sauce until it just wilts down. You may need to do this in a couple of batches if you can't fit all the spinach in the pan in one go.

NUTRITION (PER SERVING):

- Calories: 311
- Protein: 16.6g
- Carbohydrates: 38.2g
- Of which sugars: 10.7g
- Fats: 9.4g
- Of which saturates: 0.8g
- Fibre: 13.4g

High in protein and a great source of key nutrients **iron** and **zinc**, plus vitamins A, B$_6$ and K, folate, copper and manganese.

SAVOURY SNACKS

GARLIC ROASTED BROCCOLI

These are a fantastic quick snack – the flavour of roasted broccoli is totally different to when it's boiled or steamed. You can also use these as a really tasty addition to salads, or as a side dish.

TIME: 5 minutes prep + 30 minutes roasting
DIFFICULTY: easy
STORAGE: best while still warm, but also nice eaten cold if kept in the fridge for up to 3 days
SERVES: 4

1 head of broccoli, chopped into bite-size spears
1 tablespoon rapeseed oil
½ teaspoon garlic powder
a good pinch of salt and pepper

Preheat the oven to 180°C/160°C fan/350°F/gas 4. Meanwhile, rinse the broccoli spears, then pat dry with kitchen paper, as excess moisture will prevent them crisping up.

Combine the broccoli with the rapeseed oil, garlic powder, salt and pepper, then spread on a baking tray in a single layer (use two trays if necessary) and pop into the oven. Roast for 25–30 minutes, checking them every 10 minutes and tossing them around so they cook evenly. Take out once they have turned crispy around the edges.

NUTRITION:
- Calories: 56
- Protein: 2.2g
- Carbohydrates: 5.2g
- Of which sugars: 1.3g
- Fats: 3.6g
- Of which saturates: 0.3g
- Fibre: 2.0g

High in vitamins C and K.

QUICK HOMEMADE HUMMUS

Homemade hummus is proof that great-tasting food can be ridiculously quick and simple to make. This has a really nice Middle Eastern flavour that most shop-bought hummus just doesn't have. Use as a dip for your favourite vegetables, spread it in sandwiches, serve with mezze, or spoon it into your salad bowls.

TIME: 10 minutes
DIFFICULTY: easy
STORAGE: keep in the fridge for up 3 days
SERVES: 4

1 x 400g tin of chickpeas, drained
1 clove of garlic, finely chopped
1 tablespoon tahini
juice of ½ a lemon
1 tablespoon olive oil
salt and pepper
3–4 tablespoons water

Simply chuck the drained chickpeas into a food processor with the rest of the ingredients and blitz until smooth. You may need to use a spoon to scrape down the sides halfway through blitzing.

Add more water if necessary until you get the desired consistency (I find it best when it's not too thick).

NUTRITION:
- Calories: 131
- Protein: 5.2g
- Carbohydrates: 13.0g
- Of which sugars: 0.3g
- Fats: 6.4g
- Of which saturates: 0.9g
- Fibre: 2.2g

High in protein and a great source of key nutrients **iron** and **calcium**, plus vitamins B_6 and C, folate and manganese.

Flavour variation: Sun-dried tomato and basil – just add 6–8 sun-dried tomatoes, a handful of fresh basil leaves, and a tablespoon of tomato purée.

CRISPY CURRY-ROASTED CHICKPEAS

These make a great snack when you're craving a savoury treat. Rather than the 'empty calories' of a bag of crisps, these will provide some healthy fats, and important calcium, iron, and zinc. They only stay crispy for a few hours, but the slightly chewy texture they get after a day or two in the fridge is quite nice too. Great as a snack, and lovely to add some bite and protein to a salad.

TIME: 5 minutes prep + 40 minutes roasting
DIFFICULTY: easy
STORAGE: best eaten fresh but can be kept in fridge for 3 days
SERVES: 4

1 x 400g tin of chickpeas, drained and rinsed
1 tablespoon rapeseed oil
1 teaspoon curry powder
¼ teaspoon garlic powder
½ teaspoon ground cumin
a pinch of salt

Preheat the oven to 190°C/170°C fan/375°F/gas 5. Take extra care to dry the chickpeas, using a couple of sheets of kitchen paper or a clean tea towel. The drier you can make them, the crispier they will get.

Remove any skins that have fallen off the chickpeas, toss the chickpeas in the oil, spices and salt, spread them on a baking tray, and roast for up to 40 minutes, shaking the tray halfway through.

Remove from the oven once they are golden and crispy.

NUTRITION:

- Calories: 107
- Protein: 4.5g
- Carbohydrates: 11.5g
- Of which sugars: 0.2g
- Fats: 4.4g
- Of which saturates: 0.4g
- Fibre: 1.8g

High in protein and a great source of the key nutrient **iron**, plus vitamin B_6, folate and manganese.

CRISPY SRIRACHA-BAKED TOFU

I use this recipe a lot, because it's so quick and versatile, and so tasty. I often use this tofu in stir-fries, curries, salads, in burritos, sandwiches, or just on its own as a snack.

Feel free to play with the ratios a little, depending on how spicy you like it – add more sriracha for a more fiery kick, or try a touch of maple syrup if you'd like a little more sweetness.

TIME: 10 minutes prep + 30 minutes baking
DIFFICULTY: easy
STORAGE: can be kept in fridge for 3 days
SERVES: 2

1 x 280g block of extra firm tofu (this also works well with tempeh)
1½ tablespoons soy sauce (sub 1 tablespoon tamari for GF)
1½ tablespoons sriracha
1 teaspoon cornflour

Preheat the oven to 200°C/180°C fan/400°F/gas 6.

Gently squeeze the tofu block between your hands to drain off any excess liquid, then slice it into smallish cubes.

Mix the soy sauce and sriracha in a mixing bowl to combine, then gently stir the cubed tofu through the mixture. Add the cornflour and use your hands to gently toss to coat the tofu.

Place the tofu cubes on a lined baking sheet and bake for 15 minutes. Then flip them over and return them to the oven for another 10–15 minutes, until golden and crispy.

NUTRITION:

- Calories: 180
- Protein: 12.3g
- Carbohydrates: 18.7g
- Of which sugars: 2.6g
- Fats: 12.5g
- Of which saturates: 0.9g
- Fibre: 1.3g

High in protein and a great source of key nutrients **iron** and **calcium**, plus phosphorus, copper and manganese.

SPICY SEED MIX

These are so tasty – they make the perfect snack, or they can be used to top salads or soups. They keep for a long time, so make a big batch to nibble on for weeks!

TIME: 20 minutes
DIFFICULTY: easy
STORAGE: store in an airtight container for up to 3 weeks
MAKES: 10 servings

250g mixed seeds – sunflower, pumpkin, flaxseed (linseed)
1 teaspoon rapeseed oil
1 teaspoon soy sauce (sub ½ teaspoon tamari for GF option)
1 teaspoon agave syrup
½ teaspoon ground cumin
½ teaspoon chilli powder

Preheat the oven to 160°C/140°C fan/325°F/gas 3.

Mix all the ingredients together in a bowl, then spread out on a baking tray and bake for 15–20 minutes until dry and golden, stirring halfway through cooking.

NUTRITION:

- Calories: 141
- Protein: 5.4g
- Carbohydrates: 6.1
- Of which sugars: 0.8g
- Fats: 11.7g
- Of which saturates: 1.4g
- Fibre: 3.4g

High in protein and a great source of key nutrients **iron** and **omega-3**, plus vitamins E, K, riboflavin, thiamine, pantothenic acid, magnesium, phosphorus, copper and manganese.

ENERGY BALLS

These bite-size treats are so simple, but they're delicious. They have a taste and texture that's almost fudge-like, and they really help to cure any sugar cravings. They're all natural and make a perfect alternative to sweets. However, they do have a modest amount of natural sugars in them, so make these as a treat to share with friends, as 2–3 at a time should be plenty!

This is a basic recipe, so please experiment with other flavours and ingredients. They work with pretty much any type of nuts, and you can try adding cocoa powder, ground cinnamon, desiccated coconut, or other dried fruits like cranberries or apricots.

TIME: 10 minutes
DIFFICULTY: easy
STORAGE: keeps in fridge for up to 1 week
MAKES: 15 balls

1 cup of walnuts (approx. 120g)
1 cup of pitted medjool dates (approx. 150g)
½ teaspoon vanilla extract

Chuck the walnuts into a food processor (not a high-speed blender like a Nutribullet – they're too fast) and blitz until coarsely ground. Add the dates and vanilla and continue blitzing until no large pieces remain.

Roll the mixture into bite-size balls, compressing them in your hands so they are packed tight. Eat straight away, or put them into the fridge for an hour to help them firm up and become more fudge-like.

NUTRITION (PER 3 BALLS):

- Calories: 236
- Protein: 4.1g
- Carbohydrates: 25.8g
- Of which sugars: 20.6g
- Fats: 15.3g
- Of which saturates: 1.5g
- Fibre: 3.6g

High in protein and a great source of key nutrient **omega-3**, plus vitamin B_6, thiamine, folate, magnesium, potassium, copper and manganese.

POPCORN

Popcorn is the ultimate happy food – crunchy, nutty and surprisingly filling. This wholegrain snack is a nutritional powerhouse, and it's so versatile, as it takes on the flavours of anything you add to it – sweet or savoury. Two cups comes in at just 73 calories!

TIME: 5 minutes
DIFFICULTY: easy
STORAGE: keep in an airtight container for up to 3 days
MAKES: 4 cups

1 teaspoon vegetable oil
2 tablespoons corn kernels

Heat the oil in a large lidded pan over a medium-high heat, then add the kernels and stir so they're all coated in a little oil. Pop the lid on, and wait for the magic to happen! They should start popping within a couple of minutes. Shake the pan occasionally so the kernels get heated evenly, and remove from the heat when the popping slows down to one every 2–3 seconds.

NUTRITION (PER 2 CUPS):

- Calories: 73
- Protein: 1.5g
- Carbohydrates: 10.4g
- Of which sugars: 0.2g
- Fats: 2.9g
- Of which saturates: 0.3g
- Fibre: 1.8g

I love popcorn just plain, but you can have fun experimenting with different flavour combinations depending on what mood you're in! Here are some examples of flavours I like to use:

SWEET CINNAMON:
Add 1 teaspoon of ground cinnamon plus 1 teaspoon of fine caster sugar.

DARK CHOCOLATE DRIZZLE:
Melt 30g of vegan dark chocolate and drizzle it over the fresh popcorn.

SMOKEY BARBECUE:
Mix in 2 teaspoons of smoked paprika, ½ teaspoon of garlic powder, and 1 tablespoon of maple syrup.

Great source of vitamins E and K, thiamine and magnesium.

PROTEIN OAT BARS

These oat bars are the perfect post-workout fuel: high in protein for recovery, with a good mix of simple and complex carbohydrates to refuel your muscle glycogen stores.

I wanted to call these flapjacks, but because they're not made with butter and copious amounts of golden syrup they're not quite like a traditional flapjack, so I didn't want to mislead you. This version, however, is oil-free and gets its sweetness from bananas, dried fruit and just a little maple syrup. They are delicious and have a great texture, soft in the middle, chewy on the outside, with some crunch from the nuts and seeds.

TIME: 10 minutes prep + 25 minutes cooking
DIFFICULTY: easy
STORAGE: keep in the fridge for up to 3 days, or freeze for up to 3 months
MAKES: 10 bars

2 large ripe bananas
150g oats (or GF oats)
25g pumpkin seeds
25g sunflower seeds
50g walnuts, roughly chopped
80g raisins
180g smooth peanut butter
5 tablespoons maple syrup
3 tablespoons soy milk

Preheat your oven to 180°C/160°C fan/350°F/gas 4. Line a small (23cm x 23cm) baking tray with baking paper and set aside.
In a large mixing bowl, mash the bananas until they become runny. Add the oats, seeds, walnuts and raisins.

Tip the peanut butter and maple syrup into a small saucepan and heat gently to soften the peanut butter and combine. Pour the peanut butter/maple syrup mixture into the oats mixture along with the soy milk, and stir until all the dry ingredients are fully coated with the wet ingredients.

Transfer the mixture to the lined baking tray and flatten the mixture down with a spoon until level. Bake in the oven for around 25 minutes, or until just turning golden around the edges.

Allow to cool for at least 10 minutes before removing from the tin and cutting into 10 bars.

NUTRITION (PER BAR):
- Calories: 251
- Protein: 9.5g
- Carbohydrates: 31.8g
- Of which sugars: 14.5g
- Fats: 16.2g
- Of which saturates: 2.2g
- Fibre: 4.3g

High in protein and a great source of key nutrients **iron**, **zinc**, and **omega-3**, plus vitamin K, riboflavin, thiamine, magnesium, potassium, phosphorus and manganese.

TOP TIP:
Try stirring through or topping with some optional extras, for example other dried fruits, ground cinnamon, vegan chocolate chips, orange zest, sesame seeds, or other nuts and seeds. Get creative!

HOW TO COOK GRAINS AND LEGUMES

Beans

When cooking dried beans, it's usually best to soak them in water overnight first. This helps increase the protein digestibility,[1] significantly reduces cooking time, and helps to reduce gas and bloating in some people. Simply soak the beans in at least triple their volume of water for around 12 hours (e.g. 1 cup dried black beans in 3+ cups of water). Then drain and rinse the beans. Place in a large pot with plenty of water, bring to the boil, then reduce the heat to a simmer and cook for 1–3 hours (depending on the type of bean), until tender. For kidney beans, boil rapidly for at least 10 minutes before the simmering stage, to destroy toxins found in raw or undercooked beans. Drain away excess water and the beans are ready to eat or use in another recipe.

1 cup of dried beans yields about 3 cups of cooked beans.

Lentils

These don't need soaking first, but a thorough rinse to make sure they're clean of any grit or dust is a good idea. Choose the right lentil for your dish – green, brown and French lentils are earthy and hold their shape when cooked, so they are versatile for most recipes. Split red or orange lentils are lovely but tend to get a little mushy when cooked, so they are great to thicken curries, for dahls or added to soups and sauces.

After rinsing, simply place the lentils with double their volume of water (i.e. 1 cup of lentils with 2 cups of water) in a pan, bring to the boil, then reduce the heat to a gentle simmer and cook uncovered for 20–30 minutes, or until the lentils are tender (split red lentils will only take about 10–15 minutes to cook, depending on how mushy you want them). Add more water if needed to make sure the lentils are just covered.

1 cup of dried lentils yields about 2½ cups of cooked lentils.

White rice

For the perfect white rice, rinse the rice thoroughly in cold water until the water runs clear, to remove some of the starch. Then place the uncooked rice in a pan with almost double its volume of cold water (e.g. 1 cup of rice with just under 2 cups of cold water). Bring to the boil, then reduce the temperature to a very gentle simmer, cover the pan with a lid, and cook for 10 minutes. After the 10 minutes is up, turn the hob off completely, but don't take the lid off the pan! You want to keep the steam inside – it will finish cooking the rice for a final 5–10 minutes.

1 cup of uncooked rice yields around 3 cups of cooked rice.

Brown rice

Brown rice takes a little longer to cook than white rice but is just as easy. Simply rinse the amount of rice you need under cold running water, then put it into a large pan with plenty of boiling water (around 6 cups of boiling water for 1 cup of brown rice). Reduce the heat to medium to maintain a steady boil, and cook for 30 minutes. Drain off the excess cooking water, then return the hot rice to the pan. Cover the pan with a lid, and let the rice steam, off the heat, for 10 minutes.

1 cup of uncooked brown rice yields around 3 cups cooked rice.

Quinoa

Lots of people have been put off quinoa because it's turned out mushy when they cook it. This method should win you back, because it results in perfect, fluffy quinoa, which will take on the flavours of dressings and sauces.

The trick is to cook the quinoa gently, as with white rice. Rinse the quinoa under cold water, then place it in a pan with double the volume of cold water (e.g. 1 cup of quinoa with 2 cups of water). Bring the water to a boil, then put a lid on the pan and reduce the heat to a very gentle simmer. Cook for about 10 minutes, until all the water has been absorbed (it may take a little longer for larger quantities). Now, take off the heat but leave the lid on to keep the steam in for 5 minutes – this process will gently finish cooking the quinoa. Fluff up with a fork and serve.

1 cup of dried quinoa yields around 3 cups of cooked quinoa.

CONCLUSION

Reaching the end of the book, I hope you now feel well equipped to enhance your plant-based nutrition, which, alongside effective training and improvements in some other lifestyle areas, will help you bring on your A-game and dominate your sport or discipline.

You've seen how the best science shows us that well-planned plant-based diets are extremely nutrient-rich and are strongly linked with powerful health benefits. On top of that, they can support improvements in recovery from exercise, and the ability to boost performance shouldn't be underestimated. When combined with other proven sports nutrition strategies such as nutrition timing and effective fuelling techniques, the results can be truly astounding.

Plant-based nutrition needn't be complicated either. Yes, we've covered a lot of theory in this book, but that theory translates into straightforward advice and meal planning guidance that has become second nature for my clients, as I'm sure it will for you, too.

While the fundamental advice within this book is unlikely to change, the theory of some of the finer details such as new ergogenic aids may evolve or develop over time, as sports nutrition science never stands still. There are new scientific studies published every day, but I hope you now have a better instinct for distinguishing between new fad, money-spinning opportunities or misinformed writers, and sound nutrition advice that might work for you and your goals.

The underpinning message throughout this book is that a well-planned plant-based diet should be varied and flexible, which helps you to carry on these healthy habits long into the future and adapt your plan as your needs change throughout life. Nothing need be rigid, and bearing in mind the principles while keeping a relaxed approach works best – this is the most effective way to ensure your healthy plant-based diet is always enjoyable and sustainable.

Whether you're a long-standing vegan or just exploring the idea of plant-based nutrition, and whether you're an elite-level athlete or someone who simply enjoys some recreational exercise, I feel confident that the principles within this book, the same principles that have helped many world-class sportspeople, will help you flourish, too.

And in flourishing, you have a tremendous power to influence and inspire others around you to at least consider a plant-based diet too. So I hope you can use what you've learned to lead by example, and help to make the world a better place.

REFERENCES

Chapter 2: Weighing up the evidence

1 Huang, R.-Y., Huang, C.-C., Hu, F., and Chavarro, J. (2016), 'Vegetarian diets and weight reduction: a meta-analysis of randomized controlled trials', *Journal of General Internal Medicine*, 31(1), 109–116.
2 Seidelmann, S., Claggett, B., Cheng, S., Henglin, et al. (2018), 'Dietary carbohydrate intake and mortality: a prospective cohort study and meta-analysis', *The Lancet Public Health*, 3(9), E419–E428.
3 Hamilton-Reeves, J. M., Vazquez, G., Duval, S. J., Phipps, W. R., Kurzer, M. S., and Messina, M. J. (2010), 'Clinical studies show no effects of soy protein or isoflavones on reproductive hormones in men: results of a meta-analysis', *Fertility and sterility*, 94(3), 997–1007.
4 Larsson, S. C., and Orsini, N. (2014), 'Red meat and processed meat consumption and all-cause mortality: a meta-analysis', *American Journal of Epidemiology*, 179 (3), 282–9.
5 Ibid.

Chapter 3: What are the health benefits of a vegan diet?

1 Dyett, P. A., Sabaté, J., Haddad, E., Rajaram, S., and Shavlik, D. (2013), 'Vegan lifestyle behaviors. An exploration of congruence with health-related beliefs and assessed health indices', *Appetite*, 67, 119–24.
2 Heiss, S., Coffino, J., and Hormes, J. (2017), 'Eating and health behaviors in vegans compared to omnivores: dispelling common myths', *Appetite*, 118, 129–35.
3 Radnitz, C., Beezhold, B., and Dimatteo, J. (2015), 'Investigation of lifestyle choices of individuals following a vegan diet for health and ethical reasons', *Appetite*, 90, 31–6.
4 Phillips, R. L. (1975), 'Role of life-style and dietary habits in risk of cancer among seventh-day adventists', *Cancer Research* (Chicago, Ill.), 35 (11 Pt. 2), 3513.
5 World Health Organization Regional Office for Europe: Cardiovascular Disease Data and Statistics, http://www.euro.who.int/en/health-topics/noncommunicable-diseases/cardiovascular-diseases/data-and-statistics.
6 Hong, Y. M. (2010), 'Atherosclerotic cardiovascular disease beginning in childhood', *Korean Circulation Journal*, 40 (1), 1–9, https://doi.org/10.4070/kcj.2010.40.1.1.
7 Wasfy, M. M., Hutter, A. M., and Weiner, R. B. (2016), 'Sudden cardiac death in athletes', *Methodist DeBakey Cardiovascular Journal*, 12 (2), 76–80, https://doi.org/10.14797/mdcj-12-2-76.
8 The International Olympic Committee (IOC) Consensus Statement on Periodic Health Evaluation of Elite Athletes (2009), https://stillmed.olympic.org/media/Document%

20Library/OlympicOrg/IOC/Who-We-Are/Commissions/Medical-and-Scientific-Commission/EN-IOC-Consensus-Statement-on-Periodic-Health-Evaluation-of-Elite-Athletes.pdf.

9 Semsarian, C., Sweeting, J., and Ackerman, M. (2015), 'Sudden cardiac death in athletes', *British Journal of Sports Medicine*, 49 (15), 1017–23.

10 Dinu, M., Abbate, R., Gensini, G., Casini, A., and Sofi, F. (2017), 'Vegetarian, vegan diets and multiple health outcomes: a systematic review with meta-analysis of observational studies', *Critical Reviews in Food Science and Nutrition*, 57 (17), 3640–49.

11 Glenn, A. J., Viguiliouk, E., Seider, M., Boucher, B. A., Khan, T. A., Blanco Mejia, S., et al. (2019), 'Relation of vegetarian dietary patterns with major cardiovascular outcomes: a systematic review and meta-analysis of prospective cohort studies', *Frontiers in Nutrition*, 6, 80.

12 Le, L., and Sabate, J. (2014), 'Beyond meatless, the health effects of vegan diets: findings from the Adventist cohorts', *Nutrients*, 6 (6), 2131–47.

13 Ornish, D., Brown, S. E., Scherwitz, L. W., Billings, J. H., Armstrong, W. T., Ports, T. A., McLanahan, S. M., Kirkeeide, R. L., Brand, R. J., and Gould, K. L. (1990), 'Can lifestyle changes reverse coronary heart disease? The Lifestyle Heart Trial', *Lancet* (London, England), 336 (8708), 129–33.

14 Snowdon, D.A. (1998), 'Animal product consumption and mortality because of all causes combined, coronary heart disease, stroke, diabetes, and cancer in Seventh-day Adventists', *American Journal of Clinial Nutrition*, 48 (suppl): 739–48.

15 Appleby, P. N., and Key, T. J. (2016), 'The long-term health of vegetarians and vegans', *Proceedings of the Nutrition Society*, 75 (3), 287–93.

16 Key, T. J., Fraser, G. E., Thorogood, M., Appleby, P. N., et al. (1999), 'Mortality in vegetarians and nonvegetarians: detailed findings from a collaborative analysis of 5 prospective studies', *American Journal of Clinical Nutrition*, 70 (3 Suppl), 516s–524s.

17 Spence, J. D. (2016), 'Metabolic vitamin B12 deficiency: a missed opportunity to prevent dementia and stroke', *Nutrition Research*, 36 (2), 109–16.

18 Chiu, T. H. T., Chang, H.-R., Wang, L.-Y., Chang, C.-C., Lin, M.-N., and Lin, C.-L. (2020), 'Vegetarian diet and incidence of total, ischemic, and hemorrhagic stroke in 2 cohorts in Taiwan', *Neurology*, 10.1212.

19 World Health Organization Regional Office for Europe: Cancer, http://www.euro.who.int/en/health-topics/noncommunicable-diseases/cancer.

20 World Health Organization Regional Office for Europe: Cancer Data and Statistics, https://www.euro.who.int/en/health-topics/noncommunicable-diseases/cancer/data-and-statistics.

21 Dinu et al. (2017), op. cit.

22 Tantamango-Bartley, Y., Jaceldo-Siegl, K., Fan, J., and Fraser, G. (2013), 'Vegetarian diets and the incidence of cancer in a low-risk population', *Cancer Epidemiology, Biomarkers & Prevention*, 22(2), 286–94.

23 World Health Organization Regional Office for Europe: Diabetes, http://www.euro.who.int/en/health-topics/noncommunicable-diseases/diabetes/diabetes.

24 Lee, Y., and Park, K. (2017), 'Adherence to a vegetarian diet and diabetes risk: a systematic review and meta-analysis of observational studies', *Nutrients*, 9 (6), 603.

25 Tonstad, S., Butler, T., Yan, R., Fraser, G. E., 'Type of vegetarian diet, body weight, and prevalence of type 2 diabetes', *Diabetes Care*, 2009; 32:791–6. doi: 10.2337/dc08-1886.

26 Tonstad, S., Stewart, K., Oda, K., Batech, M., Herring, R. P., Fraser, G. E., 'Vegetarian diets and incidence of diabetes in the Adventist Health Study-2', *Nutr. Metab. Cardiovasc Dis.* 2013; 23 (4): 292–9. doi:10.1016/j.numecd.2011.07.004.

27 Appuhamy, J., Kebreab, E., Simon, M., Yada, R., Milligan, L., and France, J. (2014), 'Effects of diet and exercise interventions on diabetes risk factors in adults without diabetes: meta-analyses of controlled trials', *Diabetology & Metabolic Syndrome*, 6 (1), 127.

28 Regensteiner, J. G., Bauer, T. A., Reusch, J. E., Quaife, R. Y., et al. (2009), 'Cardiac dysfunction during exercise in uncomplicated type 2 diabetes, *Medicine & Science in Sports & Exercise*, 41 (5), 977–84.

29 World Alzheimer Report 2015: the global impact of dementia: an analysis of prevalence, incidence, cost and trends. Alzheimer's Disease International; 2015.

30 Grant, W. B. 'Using multicountry ecological and observational studies to determine dietary risk factors for Alzheimer's disease', *Journal of the American College of Nutrition*, 2016; 35 (5): 476 doi: 10.1080/07315724.2016.1161566.

31 Giem, P., Beeson, W., and Fraser, G. (1993), 'The incidence of dementia and intake of animal products: preliminary findings from the Adventist Health Study', *Neuroepidemiology*, 12 (1), 28–36.

32 Jiang, X., Huang, J., Song, D., Deng, R., Wei, J., and Zhang, Z. (2017), 'Increased consumption of fruit and vegetables is related to a reduced risk of cognitive impairment and dementia: meta-analysis', *Frontiers in Aging Neuroscience*, 9, 18.

33 Albanese, E., Dangour, A. D., Uauy, R., Acosta, D., Guerra, M., Guerra, S. S., et al. (2009), 'Dietary fish and meat intake and dementia in Latin America, China, and India: A 10/66 Dementia Research Group population-based study', 90 (2), 392–400.

34 Beydoun, M. A., Beydoun, H. A., Gamaldo, A. A., Teel, A., Zonderman, A. B., and Wang, Y. (2014), 'Epidemiologic studies of modifiable factors associated with cognition and dementia: systematic review and meta-analysis', *BMC Public Health*, 14 (1), 643.

35 Orlich, M., Singh, P., Sabaté, J., Jaceldo-Siegl, K., Fan, J., Knutsen, S., et al. (2013), 'Vegetarian Dietary Patterns and Mortality in Adventist Health Study 2', *JAMA Internal Medicine*, 173 (13), 1230–38.

36 Hyunju, K., Caulfield, L. E., Garcia-Larsen, V., Steffen, L. M., Coresh, J., and Rebholz, C. M. (2019), 'Plant-based diets are associated with a lower risk of incident cardiovascular disease, cardiovascular disease mortality, and all-cause mortality in a general population of middle-aged adults', *Journal of the American Heart Association*, 2019; 8: e012865.

37 Larsson, S. C., and Orsini, N. (2014), 'Red meat and processed meat consumption and all-cause mortality: a meta-analysis', *American Journal of Epidemiology*, 179 (3), 282–9.

38 Aune, D., Giovannucci, E., Boffetta, P., Fadnes, L., et al. (2017), 'Fruit and vegetable intake and the risk of cardiovascular disease, total cancer and all-cause mortality – a systematic review and dose-response meta-analysis of prospective studies', *International Journal of Epidemiology*, 46 (3), 1029–56.

39 Dinu et al. (2017), op. cit.

40 Appleby, P. N., Crowe, F. L., Bradbury, K. E., Travis, R. C., and Key, T. J. (2016), 'Mortality in vegetarians and comparable nonvegetarians in the United Kingdom', *American Journal of Clinical Nutrition*, 103 (1), 218–30.

41 Parker, H., and Vadiveloo, M. (2019), 'Diet quality of vegetarian diets compared with nonvegetarian diets: a systematic review', *Nutrition Reviews*, 77 (3), 144–60.

42 Cervantes Gracia, K., Llanas-Cornejo, D., and Husi, H. (2017), 'CVD and Oxidative Stress', *Journal of Clinical Medicine*, 6 (2), 22.

43 Reuter, S., Gupta, S. C., Chaturvedi, M. M., and Aggarwal, B. B. (2010), 'Oxidative stress, inflammation, and cancer: how are they linked?', *Free Radical Biology & Medicine*, 49(11), 1603–16.

44 Erejuwa, O. O., 'Oxidative stress in diabetes mellitus: is there a role for hypoglycemic drugs and/or antioxidants', *Oxid. Stress Dis.*, 2012: 217–46.

45 Christen, Y., 'Oxidative stress and Alzheimer disease', *American Journal of Clinical Nutrition*, 2000; 71: 621s–9s.

46 Powers, S. K., Smuder, A. J., and Judge, A. R. (2012), 'Oxidative stress and disuse muscle atrophy: cause or consequence?' *Current Opinion in Clinical Nutrition and Metabolic Care*, 15 (3), 240–45.

47 Carlsen, M. H., Halvorsen, B. L., Holte, K., et al. (2010), 'The total antioxidant content of more than 3100 foods, beverages, spices, herbs and supplements used worldwide', *Nutrition Journal*, 9, 3.

48 Ristow, M., Zarse, K., Oberbach, A., Klöting, N., Birringer, M., Kiehntopf, M., et al. (2009), 'Antioxidants prevent health-promoting effects of physical exercise in humans', *Proceedings of the National Academy of Sciences*, 106 (21), 8665–70.

49 Macpherson, H., Pipingas, A., Pase, M. P. (2013), 'Multivitamin-multimineral supplementation and mortality: a meta-analysis of randomized controlled trials', *American Journal of Clinical Nutrition*, 97, (2), 437–44.

50 Bjelakovic, G., Nikolova, D., Gluud, L. L., Simonetti, R. G., and Gluud, C. (2015), 'Antioxidant supplements for prevention of mortality in healthy participants and patients with various diseases', *São Paulo Medical Journal*, 133 (2), 164–5.

51 Schwingshackl, L., Boeing, H., Stelmach-Mardas, M., Gottschald, M., Dietrich, S., Hoffmann, G., and Chaimani, A. (2017), 'Dietary supplements and risk of cause-specific death, cardiovascular disease, and cancer: a systematic review and meta-analysis of primary prevention trials', *Advances in Nutrition* (Bethesda, Md), 8 (1), 27–39.

52 Bianconi, E., Piovesan, A., Facchin, F., Beraudi, A., Casadei, R., Frabetti, F., et al. (2013), 'An estimation of the number of cells in the human body', *Annals of Human Biology*, 40 (6), 463–71.

53 National Institutes of Health, 'NIH Human Microbiome Project defines normal bacterial makeup of the body', https://www.nih.gov/news-events/news-releases/nih-human-microbiome-project-defines-normal-bacterial-makeup-body.

54 Glick-Bauer, M. C., and Yeh, M. (2014), 'The health advantage of a vegan diet: exploring the gut microbiota connection', *Nutrients*, 6 (11), 4822–38.

55 David, L. A., Maurice, C. F., Carmody, R. N., Gootenberg, D. B., Button, J. E., Wolfe, B. E., Ling, A. V., Devlin, A. S., Varma, Y., Fischbach, M. A., et al. (2014), 'Diet rapidly and reproducibly alters the human gut microbiome', *Nature*, 505, 559–63.

56 Wong, J. M., De Souza, R. W., Kendall, C. J., Emam, A., and Jenkins, D. (2006), 'Colonic health: fermentation and short chain fatty acids', *Journal of Clinical Gastroenterology*, 40 (3), 235–43.

57 Peng, L., Li, Z., Green, R., Holzman, I., and Lin, J. (2009), 'Butyrate enhances the intestinal barrier by facilitating tight junction assembly via activation of AMP-activated protein kinase in Caco-2 cell monolayers', *Journal of Nutrition*, 139 (9), 1619–25.

58 Erios-Covian, D., Eruas-Madiedo, P., Emargolles, A., Egueimonde, M., De Los Reyes-Gavilan, C. G., and Esalazar, N. (2016), 'Intestinal short chain fatty acids and their link with diet and human health', *Frontiers in Microbiology*, 7, 185.

59 House of Commons Library: Obesity Statistics (2017). https://commonslibrary.par liament.uk/research-briefings/sno3336/#:~:text=The%20Health%20Survey%20for %20England,is%20classified%20as%20'overweight'.

60 Orlich, M., and Fraser, G. (2014), 'Vegetarian diets in the Adventist Health Study 2: a review of initial published findings', *American Journal of Clinical Nutrition*, 100, 353s.

61 Dinu et al. (2017), op. cit.

62 Huang, R.-Y., Huang, C.-C., Hu, F., and Chavarro, J. (2016), 'Vegetarian diets and weight reduction: a meta-analysis of randomized controlled trials', *Journal of General Internal Medicine*, 31 (1), 109–16.

63 Ward, M. H., Cross, A. J., Abnet, C. C., Sinha, R. S., Markin, R. D., and Weisen-burger, D. (2012), 'Heme iron from meat and risk of adenocarcinoma of the esophagus and stomach', *European Journal of Cancer Prevention*, 21 (2), 134–8.

64 Bastide, N., Pierre, F., and Corpet, D. (2011), 'Heme iron from meat and risk of colorectal cancer: a meta-analysis and a review of the mechanisms involved', *Cancer Prevention Research*, 1–16.

65 Lunn, J., Kuhnle, G., Mai, V., Frankenfeld, C., Shuker, D., Glen, R., et al. (2006), 'The effect of haem in red and processed meat on the endogenous formation of N-nitroso compounds in the upper gastrointestinal tract', *Carcinogenesis*, 28 (3), 685–90.

66 Chang, V. C., Cotterchio, M., Bondy, S. J., and Kotsopoulos, J. (2020), 'Iron intake, oxidative stress-related genes, and breast cancer risk', *International Journal of Cancer*, 147 (5), 1354–73.

67 Tricker, A. R., and Preussmann, R. (1991), 'Carcinogenic N-nitrosamines in the diet: occurrence, formation, mechanisms and carcinogenic potential', *Mutation Research*, 259 (3–4), 277–89.

68 Song, P., Wu, L., and Guan, W. (2015), 'Dietary nitrates, nitrites, and nitrosamines intake and the risk of gastric cancer: a meta-analysis', *Nutrients*, 7 (12), 9872–95.

69 Cantwell, M., Elliott, C. (2017), 'Nitrates, nitrites and nitrosamines from processed meat intake and colorectal cancer risk', *Journal of Clinical Nutrition and Dietetics*, 3:27. doi: 10.4172/2472-1921.100062.

70 WHO International Agency for Research on Cancer (2015), Q&A on the carcino-genicity of the consumption of red meat and processed meat. Accessed 11.10.17 at: https://www.iarc.fr/en/media-centre/iarcnews/pdf/Monographs-Q&A_Vol114. pdf.

71 Janeiro, M., Ramírez, M., Milagro, F., Martínez, J., and Solas, M. (2018), 'Implica-tion of trimethylamine N-oxide (TMAO) in disease: potential biomarker or new therapeutic target', *Nutrients*, 10 (10).

72 Qi, J., You, T., Li, J., et al. (2018), 'Circulating trimethylamine N-oxide and the risk of cardiovascular diseases: a systematic review and meta-analysis of 11 prospective cohort studies', *Journal of Cellular and Molecular Medicine*, 22, 185–94. 10.1111/jcmm. 13307.

73 Zhuang, R., Ge, X., Han, L., Yu, P., Gong, X., Meng, Q., et al. (2019), 'Gut microbe-generated metabolite trimethylamine N-oxide and the risk of diabetes: a systematic review and dose-response meta-analysis', *Obesity Reviews*, 20 (6), 883–94.

74 Vogt, N. M., Romano, K. A., Darst, B. F., Engelman, C. D. Johnson, S. C., Carlsson, C. M., et al. (2018), 'The gut microbiota-derived metabolite trimethyl-amine N-oxide is elevated in Alzheimer's disease', *Alzheimer's Research & Therapy*, 10, Article 124.

75 Qi et al. (2018), op. cit.

76 Siri-Tarino, P., Sun, Q., Hu, F., and Krauss, R. (2010), 'Meta-analysis of prospective cohort studies evaluating the association of saturated fat with cardiovascular disease', *American Journal of Clinical Nutrition*, 91 (3), 535–46.

77 Clarke, R., Frost, C., Collins, R., Appleby, P., and Peto, R. (1997), 'Dietary lipids and blood cholesterol: quantitative meta-analysis of metabolic ward studies', *British Medical Journal*, 314 (7074), 112–17.

78 Hooper, L., Martin, N., Abdelhamid, A., and Davey Smith, G. (2015), 'Reduction in saturated fat intake for cardiovascular disease', *The Cochrane Database of Systematic Reviews*, (6), CD011737.

79 Rocha, D., Bressan, J., and Hermsdorff, H. (2017), 'The role of dietary fatty acid intake in inflammatory gene expression: a critical review', *Sao Paulo Medical Journal*, 135 (2), 157–68.

80 Späh, F. (2008), 'Inflammation in atherosclerosis and psoriasis: common pathogenic mechanisms and the potential for an integrated treatment approach', *British Journal of Dermatology*, 159, Suppl 2, 10–17.

81 Wolters, M., Ahrens, J., Romaní-Pérez, M., Watkins, C., Sanz, Y., Benítez-Páez, A., Stanton, C., and Günther, K. (2019), 'Dietary fat, the gut microbiota, and metabolic health – a systematic review conducted within the MyNewGut project', *Clinical Nutrition* (Edinburgh, Scotland), 38 (6), 2504–20.

82 Cross, A., and Sinha, R. (2004), 'Meat-related mutagens/carcinogens in the etiology of colorectal cancer', *Environmental and Molecular Mutagenesis*, 44 (1), 44–55.

83 Chiavarini, M., Bertarelli, G., Minelli, L., and Fabiani, R. (2017), 'Dietary intake of meat cooking-related mutagens (HCAs) and risk of colorectal adenoma and cancer: a systematic review and meta-analysis', *Nutrients*, 9 (5), 514.

84 Falowo, A. B., and Akimoladun, O. F. (2019), 'Veterinary Drug Residues in Meat and Meat Products: Occurrence, Detection and Implications', *Veterinary Pharmaceuticals*, IntechOpen, 1–18.

85 Murphy, N., Knuppel, A., Papadimitriou, N., Martin, R. M., Tsilidis, K. K., Smith-Byrne, K., et al. (2020), 'Insulin-like growth factor-1, insulin-like growth factor-binding protein-3, and breast cancer risk: observational and Mendelian randomization analyses with ~430 000 women', *Annals of Oncology*, 31 (5), 641–9.

86 Harrison, S., Lennon, R., Holly, J., Higgins, J., Gardner, P., Perks, T., et al. (2017), 'Does milk intake promote prostate cancer initiation or progression via effects on insulin-like growth factors (IGFs)? A systematic review and meta-analysis', *Cancer Causes & Control*, 28 (6), 497–528.

Chapter 4: Are vegans more prone to nutritional deficiencies?

1 British Nutrition Foundation: Nutrition Requirements (2019), https://www.nutrition.org.uk/attachments/article/261/Nutrition%20Requirements_Revised%20August%202019.pdf.

2 Food Standards Agency (2018), Food Supplements Consumer Research: https://www.food.gov.uk/sites/default/files/media/document/food-supplements-full-report-final-2505018.pdf.

3 Jovanov, P., Đorđić, V., Obradović, B., Barak, O., Pezo, L., Marić, A., and Sakač, M. (2019), 'Prevalence, knowledge and attitudes towards using sports supplements among young athletes', *Journal of the International Society of Sports Nutrition*, 16 (1), 27.

4 British Dietetic Association: Fibre Food Fact Sheet, https://www.bda.uk.com/resource/fibre.html#:~:text=In%20the%20UK%2C%20the%20average,try%20to%20eat%20g%20more.

5 Clarys, P., Deliens, T., Huybrechts, I., Deriemaeker, P., et al. (2014), 'Comparison of nutritional quality of the vegan, vegetarian, semi-vegetarian, pesco-vegetarian and omnivorous diet', *Nutrients*, 6 (3), 1318–32.

6 Rizzo, N. S., Jaceldo-Siegl, K., Sabate, J., and Fraser, G. E. (2013), 'Nutrient profiles of vegetarian and nonvegetarian dietary patterns', *Journal of the Academy of Nutrition and Dietetics*, 113 (12), 1610–19, https://doi.org/10.1016/j.jand.2013.06.349

7 McRae, M. P. (2017), 'Dietary fiber is beneficial for the prevention of cardiovascular disease: an umbrella review of meta-analyses', *Journal of Chiropractic Medicine*, 16 (4), 289–99.

8 Manach, C., Williamson, G., Morand, C., Scalbert, A., Remesy, C. (2005), 'Bioavailability and bioefficacy of polyphenols in humans. I. Review of 97 bioavailability studies', *American Journal of Clinical Nutrition*, 81 (1), 230S–42S.

9 Cömert, E. D., and Gökmen, V. (2017), 'Antioxidants bound to an insoluble food matrix: their analysis, regeneration behavior, and physiological importance', *Comprehensive Reviews in Food Science and Food Safety*, 16, 382–99.

10 Smith, J. A. (1995), 'Exercise, training and red blood cell turnover', *Sports Medicine* (Auckland, NZ), 19 (1), 9–31.

11 NHS: Vitamins, Supplements and Nutrition in Pregnancy, https://www.nhs.uk/conditions/pregnancy-and-baby/vitamins-minerals-supplements-pregnant/.

12 British Nutrition Foundation: Summary of Key Findings from the NDNS Report of Years 7&8 (Combined), https://www.nutrition.org.uk/nutritioninthenews/newreports/ndnsyears7and8.html.

13 Gilsing, A. M. J., Crowe, F. L., Lloyd-Wright, Z., Sanders, T. A. B., Appleby, P. N., Allen, N. E., and Key, T. J. (2010), 'Serum concentrations of vitamin B12 and folate in British male omnivores, vegetarians and vegans: Results from a cross-sectional analysis of the EPIC-Oxford cohort study', *European Journal of Clinical Nutrition*, 64 (9), 933–9.

14 Harvard Health Publishing: Potassium and Sodium out of Balance, https://www.health.harvard.edu/staying-healthy/potassium_and_sodium_out_of_balance.

15 Aburto, N., Hanson, S., Gutierrez, H., Hooper, L., Elliott, P., and Cappuccio, F. (2013). 'Effect of increased potassium intake on cardiovascular risk factors and disease: systematic review and meta-analyses', *British Medical Journal*, 346 (3), F1378.

16 Lennon-Edwards, S., Allman, B., Schellhardt, T., Ferreira, C., Farquhar, W., and Edwards, D. (2014), 'Lower potassium intake is associated with increased wave reflection in young healthy adults', *Nutrition Journal*, 13 (1), 39.

17 Lambert, H., Boyd, V., Darling, A., Torgerson, D., Burckhardt, P., Frassetto, L., and Lanham-New, S. (2011), 'Evidence for the role of potassium in bone health: results of a systematic review and meta-analysis', *Proceedings of the Nutrition Society, 70* (OCE3), E86–E86.

18 Roberts, C., Steer, T., Maplethorpe, N., Cox, L., Meadows, S., et al. (2018), National Diet and Nutrition Survey: Results from Years 7 and 8 (combined) of the Rolling Programme (2014/2015–2015/2016).

19 Cogswell, M. E., Zhang, Z., Carriquiry, A. L., Gunn, J. P., Kuklina, E. V., et al. (2012), 'Sodium and potassium intakes among US adults: NHANES 2003–2008', *American Journal of Clinical Nutrition*, 96 (3), 647–57.

20 Rizzo et al. (2013), op. cit.

21 Nielsen, F. H. (2018), 'Magnesium deficiency and increased inflammation: current perspectives', *Journal of Inflammation Research*, 11, 25–34. 10.2147/JIR.S136742.

22 Ryder, K., Shorr, R., Bush, A., Kritchevsky, S., Harris, T., et al. (2005), 'Magnesium intake from food and supplements is associated with bone mineral density in healthy older white subjects', *Journal of the American Geriatrics Society*, 53 (11), 1875–80.

23 Derbyshire, E. (2018), 'Micronutrient intakes of British adults across mid-life: a secondary analysis of the UK National Diet and Nutrition Survey', *Frontiers in Nutrition* (Lausanne), 5, 55.

24 Nielsen, F., and Lukaski, H. (2006), 'Update on the relationship between magnesium and exercise', *Magnesium research: official organ of the International Society for the Development of Research on Magnesium*, 19, 180–89.

25 Davey, G., Spencer, E., Appleby, P., Allen, N., Knox, K., and Key, T. (2003), 'EPIC–Oxford: lifestyle characteristics and nutrient intakes in a cohort of 33 883 meat-eaters and 31 546 non meat-eaters in the UK', *Public Health Nutrition*, 6 (3), 259–68.

26 Rizzo et al., (2013), op. cit.

Chapter 5: Key nutrients for vegans

1 Ma, Y., Peng, D., Liu, C., Huang, C., and Luo, J. (2017), 'Serum high concentrations of homocysteine and low levels of folic acid and vitamin B12 are significantly correlated with the categories of coronary artery diseases', *BMC Cardiovascular Disorders*, 17(1).

2 Fan, R., Zhang, A., and Zhong, F. (2017), 'Association between homocysteine levels and all-cause mortality: a dose-response meta-analysis of prospective studies', *Scientific Reports*, 7 (1), 4769.

3 Gilsing, A. M., Crowe, F. L., Lloyd-Wright, Z., Sanders, T. A., Appleby, P. N., Allen, N. E., and Key, T. J. (2010), 'Serum concentrations of vitamin B12 and folate in British male omnivores, vegetarians and vegans: results from a cross-sectional analysis of the EPIC-Oxford cohort study', *European Journal of Clinical Nutrition*, 64 (9), 933–9.

4 Pawlak, R., Lester, S. E., and Babatunde, T. (2014), 'The prevalence of cobalamin deficiency among vegetarians assessed by serum vitamin B12: A review of literature', *European Journal of Clinical Nutrition*, 68 (5), 541–8.

5 The Vegan Society: Vitamin B12. https://www.vegansociety.com/resources/nutrition-and-health/nutrients/vitamin-b12.

6 British Dietetic Association: Nutritional Considerations for Dietitians. Vitamin B12. https://www.bda.uk.com/uploads/assets/3305b792-a139-4ab8-bbecdd5dc7f2cbf9/Practical-guide-nutritional-considerations-VITAMIN-B12.pdf.

7 Scientific Advisory Committee on Nutrition: Iron and Health. https://assets.publishing.service.gov.uk/government/uploads/system/uploads/attachment_data/file/339309/SACN_Iron_and_Health_Report.pdf.

8 Davey, G., Spencer, E., Appleby, P., Allen, N., Knox, K., and Key, T. (2003), 'EPIC–Oxford: lifestyle characteristics and nutrient intakes in a cohort of 33 883 meat-eaters and 31 546 non meat-eaters in the UK, *Public Health Nutrition*, 6 (3), 259–68.

9 Haider, L., Schwingshackl, L., Hoffmann, G., and Ekmekcioglu, C. (2018), 'The effect of vegetarian diets on iron status in adults: A systematic review and meta-analysis', *Critical Reviews in Food Science and Nutrition*, 58 (8), 1359–74.

10 Monsen, E. R. (1988), 'Iron nutrition and absorption: dietary factors which impact iron bioavailability', *Journal of the American Dietetic Association*, 88 (7), 786–90.

11 Salovaara, S., Sandberg, A., and Andlid, T. (2002), 'Organic acids influence iron uptake in the human epithelial cell line Caco-2', *Journal of Agricultural and Food Chemistry*, 50 (21), 6233–8.

12 Aune, D., Chan, D., Lau, R., Vieira, R., Greenwood, D., Kampman, E., and Norat, T. (2011), 'Dietary fibre, whole grains, and risk of colorectal cancer: systematic review and dose-response meta-analysis of prospective studies', *British Medical Journal*, 343 (7833), D6617.

13 Slavin, J. L. (2000), 'Mechanisms for the impact of whole grain foods on cancer risk', *Journal of the American College of Nutrition*, 19 (3 Suppl), 300s–307s.

14 Siegenberg, D., Baynes, R. D., Bothwell, T. H., et al. (1991), 'Ascorbic acid prevents the dose-dependent inhibitory effects of polyphenols and phytates on nonheme-iron absorption', *American Journal of Clinical Nutrition*, 53 (2), 537–41.

15 Foster, M., Chu, A., Petocz, P., and Samman, S. (2013), 'Effect of vegetarian diets on zinc status: a systematic review and meta-analysis of studies in humans', *Journal of the Science of Food and Agriculture*, 93 (10), 2362–71.

16 Micheletti, A., Rossi, R., and Rufini, S. (2001), 'Zinc status in athletes: Relation to diet and exercise', *Sports Medicine* (Auckland, NZ), 31 (8), 577–82.

17 Institute of Medicine (US) Panel on Micronutrients (2001), *Dietary Reference Intakes for Vitamin A, Vitamin K, Arsenic, Boron, Chromium, Copper, Iodine, Iron, Manganese, Molybdenum, Nickel, Silicon, Vanadium, and Zinc*, Washington (DC): National Academies Press (US), 12, Zinc. Available from: https://www.ncbi.nlm.nih.gov/books/NBK222317/.

18 Gautam, S., Platel, K., and Srinivasan, K. (2010), 'Higher bioaccessibility of iron and zinc from food grains in the presence of garlic and onion', *Journal of Agricultural and Food Chemistry*, 58 (14), 8426–9.

19 Simopoulos, A. (2006), 'Evolutionary aspects of diet, the omega-6/omega-3 ratio and genetic variation: nutritional implications for chronic diseases', *Biomedicine & Pharmacotherapy*, 60 (9), 502–7.

20 Simopoulos, A. (2008), 'The Importance of the Omega-6/Omega-3 Fatty Acid Ratio in Cardiovascular Disease and Other Chronic Diseases', *Experimental Biology and Medicine*, 233 (6), 674–88.

21 Burdge, G. (2004), 'Alpha-linolenic acid metabolism in men and women: nutritional and biological implications', *Current Opinion in Clinical Nutrition and Metabolic Care*, 7 (2), 137–44.

22 Rosell, M., Lloyd-Wright, Z., Appleby, P., Sanders, T., Allen, N., and Key, T. (2005), 'Long-chain n-3 polyunsaturated fatty acids in plasma in British meat-eating, vegetarian, and vegan men', *American Journal of Clinical Nutrition*, 82 (2), 327–34.

23 Liou, Y. A., King, D. J., Zibrik, D., and Innis, S. M. (2007), 'Decreasing linoleic acid with constant α-linolenic acid in dietary fats increases (n-3) eicosapentaenoic acid in plasma phospholipids in healthy men', *Journal of Nutrition*, 137 (4), 945–52.

24 NHS: The Eatwell Guide, https://www.nhs.uk/live-well/eat-well/the-eatwell-guide/.

25 European Food Safety Authority: Daily Reference Values for the EU, http://www.efsa.europa.eu/en/interactive-pages/drvs.

26 Masley, S., Masley, L., and Gualtieri, C. (2012), 'Effect of mercury levels and seafood intake on cognitive function in middle-aged adults', *Integrative Medicine*, 11 (3), 32–40.

27 Bourdon, J., Bazinet, T., Arnason, T., Kimpe, L., Blais, J., and White, P. (2010), 'Polychlorinated biphenyls (PCBs) contamination and aryl hydrocarbon receptor (AhR) agonist activity of Omega-3 polyunsaturated fatty acid supplements:

Implications for daily intake of dioxins and PCBs', *Food and Chemical Toxicology*, 48 (11), 3093–7.

28 Bernstein, A. M., Ding, E. L., Willett, W. C., Rimm, E. B. (2012), 'A meta-analysis shows that docosahexaenoic acid from algal oil reduces serum triglycerides and increases HDL-cholesterol and LDL-cholesterol in persons without coronary heart disease', *Journal of Nutrition*, 142 (1), 99–104.

29 Ryan, L., and Symington, A. (2015), 'Algal-oil supplements are a viable alternative to fish-oil supplements in terms of docosahexaenoic acid (22:6n-3; DHA)', *Journal of Functional Foods*, 19, 852–8.

30 Ryan, A. S., Keske, M. A., Hoffman, J. P., and Nelson, E. B. (2009), 'Clinical overview of algal-docosahexaenoic acid: effects on triglyceride levels and other cardiovascular risk factors', *American Journal of Therapeutics*, 16 (2), 183–92.

31 Robertson, R. C., Guihéneuf, F., Bahar, B., Schmid, M., Stengel, D. B., Fitzgerald, G. F., Ross, R. P., and Stanton, C. (2015), 'The anti-inflammatory effect of algae-derived lipid extracts on lipopolysaccharide (LPS)-stimulated human THP-1 macrophages', *Marine Drugs*, 13 (8), 5402–24, https://doi.org/10.3390/md13085402.

32 Mickleborough, T. (2013), 'Omega-3 polyunsaturated fatty acids in physical performance optimization', *International Journal of Sport Nutrition and Exercise Metabolism*, 23 (1), 83–96.

33 Lv, Z., Zhang, J., and Zhu, W. (2020), 'Omega-3 polyunsaturated fatty acid supplementation for reducing muscle soreness after eccentric exercise: a systematic review and meta-analysis of randomized controlled trials', *BioMed Research International*, 2020, 8062017.

34 Rossato, L., Schoenfeld, B., and De Oliveira, E. (2020), 'Is there sufficient evidence to supplement omega-3 fatty acids to increase muscle mass and strength in young and older adults?', *Clinical Nutrition*, 39 (1), 23–32.

35 Tenforde, Adam, Sayres, Lauren, Sainani, Kristin, and Fredericson, Michael (2010), 'Evaluating the relationship of calcium and vitamin D in the prevention of stress fracture injuries in the young athlete: a review of the literature', *PM & R: The Journal of Injury, Function, and Rehabilitation*, 2. 945-9. 10.1016/j.pmrj.2010.05.006.

36 Office of the Surgeon General (US), 'Bone Health and Osteoporosis: A Report of the Surgeon General', Rockville (MD): Office of the Surgeon General (US); 2004. 6, Determinants of Bone Health. Available from: https://www.ncbi.nlm.nih.gov/books/NBK45503/.

37 Hilliard, Constance B. (2016), 'High osteoporosis risk among East Africans linked to lactase persistence genotype', BoneKEy Reports, 5, 803.

38 British Nutrition Foundation: Dietary Calcium and Health, https://www.nutrition.org.uk/attachments/205_Dietary%20calcium%20and%20health%20summary.pdf.

39 Clarys, P., Deliens, T., Huybrechts, I., Deriemaeker, P., Vanaelst, B., De Keyzer, W., Hebbelinck, M., and Mullie, P. (2014), 'Comparison of nutritional quality of the vegan, vegetarian, semi-vegetarian, pesco-vegetarian and omnivorous diet', *Nutrients*, 6 (3), 1318–32.

40 Iguacel, I., Miguel-Berges, M., Gómez-Bruton, A., Moreno, L., and Julián, C. (2019), 'Veganism, vegetarianism, bone mineral density, and fracture risk: a systematic review and meta-analysis', *Nutrition Reviews*, 77 (1), 1–18.

41 Appleby, P., Roddam, A., Allen, N., and Key, T. (2007), 'Comparative fracture risk in vegetarians and nonvegetarians in EPIC–Oxford', *European Journal of Clinical Nutrition*, 61 (12), 1400–1406.

42 Weaver C. M., Plawecki, K. L. (1994), 'Dietary calcium: adequacy of a vegetarian diet', *American Journal of Clinical Nutrition*, 59 (5 Suppl), 1238s–1241s.

43 Barzel, U. S., and Massey, L. K. (1998), 'Excess dietary protein can adversely affect bone', *Journal of Nutrition*, 128, 1051–3.

44 Kerstetter, J. E., O'Brien, K. O., Caseria, D. M., Wall, D. E., and Insogna, K. L. (2005), 'The impact of dietary protein on calcium absorption and kinetic measures of bone turnover in women', *The Journal of Clinical Endocrinology and Metabolism*, 90 (1), 26–31.

45 Cao, J. J., Johnson, L. K., and Hunt, J. R. (2011), 'A diet high in meat protein and potential renal acid load increases fractional calcium absorption and urinary calcium excretion without affecting markers of bone resorption or formation in postmenopausal women', *Journal of Nutrition*, 141 (3), 391–7.

46 Maalouf, N. M., Moe, O. W., Adams-Huet, B., and Sakhaee, K. (2011), 'Hypercalciuria associated with high dietary protein intake is not due to acid load', *Journal of Clinical Endocrinology and Metabolism*, 96 (12), 3733–40.

47 Heaney, R., Dowell, M., Hale, C., and Bendich, A. (2003), 'Calcium absorption varies within the reference range for serum 25-hydroxyvitamin D', *Journal of the American College of Nutrition*, 22 (2), 142–6.

48 Holick, M. F. (2007), 'Vitamin D deficiency', *New England Journal of Medicine*, 357 (3), 266–81.

49 Crowe, F. L., Steur, M., Allen, N. E., Appleby, P. N., Travis, R. C., and Key, T. J. (2011), 'Plasma concentrations of 25-hydroxyvitamin D in meat eaters, fish eaters, vegetarians and vegans: results from the EPIC–Oxford study', *Public Health Nutrition*, 14 (2), pp.340–46.

50 Chan, J., Jaceldo-Siegl, K., and Fraser, G. E. (2009), 'Serum 25-hydroxyvitamin D status of vegetarians, partial vegetarians, and nonvegetarians: the Adventist Health Study-2', *American Journal of Clinical Nutrition*, 89 (5), 1686S–1692S.

51 Bates, B., Lennox, A., Prentice, A., Bates, C., Page, P., Nicholson, S. and Swan, G. (2014), 'The National Diet and Nutrition Survey: Results from Years 1, 2, 3 and 4 (combined) of the Rolling Programme (2008/2009 – 2011/2012)', London: TSO.

52 Hossein-Nezhad, A., and Holick, M. (2013), 'Vitamin D for health: a global perspective', Mayo Clinic Proceedings, 88 (7), 720–55.

53 Dao, D., Sodhi, S., Tabasinejad, R., Peterson, D., Ayeni, O. R., Bhandari, M., Farrokhyar, F. (2015), 'Serum 25-hydroxyvitamin D levels and stress fractures in military personnel: a systematic review and meta-analysis', *American Journal of Sports Medicine*, 43 (8), 2064–72. Epub 2014 Nov 4.

54 Williams, K., Askew, C., Mazoue, C., Guy, J., Torres-McGehee, T. M., and Jackson III, J. B. (2020), 'Vitamin D3 supplementation and stress fractures in high-risk collegiate athletes – a pilot study', *Orthopedic Research and Reviews*, 12, 9–17.

55 Public Health England: PHE Published New Advice on Vitamin D, https://www.gov.uk/government/news/phe-publishes-new-advice-on-vitamin-d.

56 NHS: How to get Vitamin D from sunlight, https://www.nhs.uk/live-well/healthy-body/how-to-get-vitamin-d-from-sunlight/.

57 National Institute for Health and Care Excellence: Sunlight Exposure: Risks and Benefits, https://www.nice.org.uk/guidance/ng34/chapter/supporting-information-for-practitioners.

58 Tripkovic, L., Lambert, H., Hart, K., et al. (2012), 'Comparison of vitamin D2 and vitamin D3 supplementation in raising serum 25-hydroxyvitamin D status: a systematic review and meta-analysis', *American Journal of Clinical Nutrition*, 95 (6), 1357–64.

59 Smyth, P. P., and Duntas, L. H. (2005), 'Iodine uptake and loss – can frequent strenuous exercise induce iodine deficiency?', *Hormone and Metabolic Research,* 37 (9), 555–8.

60 Biban, B. G., and Lichiardopol, C. (2017), 'Iodine deficiency, still a global problem?', *Current Health Sciences Journal,* 43 (2), pp.103–11.

61 World Health Organization: Iodine Deficiency Disorders, https://www.who.int/nutrition/topics/idd/en/.

62 Food Standards Agency and Public Health England: NDNS: Results from Years 7 & 8 (Combined), https://www.gov.uk/government/statistics/ndns-results-from-years-7-and-8-combined.

63 Sobiecki, J. G., Appleby, P. N., Bradbury, K. E., Key, T. J. (2016), 'High compliance with dietary recommendations in a cohort of meat eaters, fish eaters, vegetarians, and vegans: results from the European Prospective Investigation into Cancer and Nutrition–Oxford study', *Nutrition Research,* 36 (5), 464–77.

64 Fuge, R. (1996), 'Geochemistry of iodine in relation to iodine deficiency diseases', Geological Society, London, Special Publications, 113, 201.

65 Zimmermann, M. B. (2009), 'Iodine deficiency', *Endocrine Reviews,* 30 (4), 376–408.

66 British Dietetic Association: Iodine Food Fact Sheet. https://www.bda.uk.com/uploads/assets/4097b9d9-1018-4dfe-aaee8d6b3205e08b/Iodine-food-fact-sheet.pdf.

67 ibid.

68 Phillips, D. I. (1997), 'Iodine, milk, and the elimination of endemic goitre in Britain: the story of an accidental public health triumph', *Journal of Epidemiology and Community Health,* 51, 391–3.

69 Atkins, P. (2005), 'The milk in schools scheme, 1934–45: "nationalization" and resistance', *History of Education,* 34 (1), 1–21.

70 Fan, Y. (2020), 'Circulating selenium and cardiovascular or all-cause mortality in the general population: a meta-analysis', *Biological Trace Element Research,* 195 (1), 55–62.

71 Rayman, M. P. (2019), 'Multiple nutritional factors and thyroid disease, with particular reference to autoimmune thyroid disease', *Proceedings of the Nutrition Society,* 78, 34–44.

72 Avery, J. C., and Hoffmann, P. R. (2018), 'Selenium, selenoproteins, and immunity', *Nutrients,* 10 (9), 1203.

73 Hurst, R., Hooper, L., Norat, T., Lau, R., Aune, D., Greenwood, D., et al. (2012), 'Selenium and prostate cancer: systematic review and meta-analysis', *American Journal of Clinical Nutrition,* 96 (1), 111–22.

74 Cai, X., Wang, C., Yu, W., Fan, W., et al. (2016), 'Selenium exposure and cancer risk: an updated meta-analysis and meta-regression', *Scientific Reports,* 6 (1), 19213.

75 Zhang, X., Liu, C., Guo, J., and Song, Y. (2015), 'Selenium status and cardiovascular diseases: meta-analysis of prospective observational studies and randomized controlled trials', *European Journal of Clinical Nutrition,* 70 (2), 162–9.

76 Wang, X., Yang, T., Wei, J., Lei, G., and Zeng, C. (2016), 'Association between serum selenium level and type 2 diabetes mellitus: a non-linear dose-response meta-analysis of observational studies', *Nutrition Journal,* 15 (1), 48.

77 Expert Group on Vitamins and Minerals 2003, Safe Upper Levels for Vitamins and Minerals, Food Standards Agency.

78 Scientific Advisory Committee on Nutrition: SACN Position Statement on Selenium and Health. https://assets.publishing.service.gov.uk/government/uploads/system/uploads/attachment_data/file/339431/SACN_Selenium_and_Health_2013.pdf

79 Sobiecki, J. (2017), 'Vegetarianism and colorectal cancer risk in a low-selenium environment: effect modification by selenium status? A possible factor contributing to the null results in British vegetarians', *European Journal of Nutrition,* 56 (5), 1819–32.

80 Parekha, P. P., Khana, A. R., Torresa, M. A., and Kitto, M. E. (2008), 'Concentrations of selenium, barium, and radium in Brazil nuts', *Journal of Food Composition and Analysis*, 21 (4), 332–5.

81 Pacheco, A. M., and Scussel, V. M. (2007), 'Selenium and aflatoxin levels in raw Brazil nuts from the Amazon basin', *Journal of Agricultural and Food Chemistry*, 55 (26), 11087–92.

82 Silva Junior, E. C., Wadt, L. H. O., Silva, K. E., Lima, R. M. B., Batista, K. D, Guedes, M. C., et al. (2017), 'Natural variation of selenium in Brazil nuts and soils from the Amazon region', *Chemosphere*, 188, 650–58.

83 Thomson, C. D., Chisholm, A., McLachlan, S. K., and Campbell, J. M. (2008), 'Brazil nuts: an effective way to improve selenium status', *American Journal of Clinical Nutrition*, 87 (2), 379–84.

Chapter 6: Recovery

1 Kawamura, T., and Muraoka, I. (2018), 'Exercise-induced oxidative stress and the effects of antioxidant intake from a physiological viewpoint', *Antioxidants*, 7 (9), 119.

2 Mastaloudis, A., Yu, T., O'Donnell, R., Frei, B., Dashwood, R., and Traber, M. (2004), 'Endurance exercise results in DNA damage as detected by the comet assay', *Free Radical Biology and Medicine*, 36 (8), 966–75.

3 ibid.

4 Sousa, C., Sales, V., Rosa, M., Lewis, M., Andrade, T., and Simões, S. (2017), 'The antioxidant effect of exercise: a systematic review and meta-analysis', *Sports Medicine*, 47 (2), 277–93.

5 Tryfidou, D., McClean, C., Nikolaidis, M., and Davison, G. (2020), 'DNA damage following acute aerobic exercise: a systematic review and meta-analysis', *Sports Medicine* (Auckland, NZ), 50 (1), 103–27.

6 Ristow, M., Zarse, K., Oberbach, A., Klöting, N., et al. (2009), 'Antioxidants prevent health-promoting effects of physical exercise in humans', *Proceedings of the National Academy of Sciences*, 106 (21), 8665–70.

7 Childs, A., Jacobs, C., Kaminski, T., Halliwell, B., and Leeuwenburgh, C. (2001), 'Supplementation with vitamin C and N-acetyl-cysteine increases oxidative stress in humans after an acute muscle injury induced by eccentric exercise', *Free Radical Biology and Medicine*, 31 (6), 745–53.

8 McAnulty, S. R., McAnulty, L. S., Nieman, D. C., Dumke, C. L., Morrow, J. D., Utter, A. C., et al. (2004), 'Consumption of blueberry polyphenols reduces exercise-induced oxidative stress compared to vitamin C', *Nutrition Research*, 24 (3), 209–21. doi: 10.1016/j.nutres.2003.10.003.

9 Chang, W. H., Hu, S. P., Huang, Y. F., Yeh, T. S., Liu, J. F. (2010), 'Effect of purple sweet potato leaves consumption on exercise-induced oxidative stress and IL-6 and HSP72 levels', *Journal of Applied Physiology*, 109 (6), 1710–15.

10 Fogarty, M. C., Hughes, C. M., Burke, G., Brown, J. C., Davison, G. W. (2013), 'Acute and chronic watercress supplementation attenuates exercise-induced peripheral mononuclear cell DNA damage and lipid peroxidation', *British Journal of Nutrition*, 109 (2), 293–301.

11 Bohlooli, S., Barmaki, S., Khoshkhahesh, F., Nakhostin-Roohi, B. (2015), 'The effect of spinach supplementation on exercise-induced oxidative stress', *Journal of Sports Medicine and Physical Fitness*, 55 (6), 609–14.

12 Mcleay, Y., Barnes, M., Mundel, T., Hurst, S., Hurst, R., and Stannard, S. (2012), 'Effect of New Zealand blueberry consumption on recovery from eccentric exercise-induced muscle damage', *Journal of the International Society of Sports Nutrition*, 9 (1), 19.

13 Lyall, K. A., Hurst, S. M., Cooney, J., Jensen, D., Lo, K., Hurst, R. D., and Stevenson, L. M. (2009), 'Short-term blackcurrant extract consumption modulates exercise-induced oxidative stress and lipopolysaccharide-stimulated inflammatory responses', *American Journal of Physiology – Regulatory, Integrative and Comparative Physiology*, 297 (1), R70–R81.

14 Funes, L., Carrera-Quintanar, L., Cerdán-Calero, M., Ferrer, M. D., Drobnic, F., Pons, A., Roche, E., and Micol, V. (2011), 'Effect of lemon verbena supplementation on muscular damage markers, proinflammatory cytokines release and neutrophils' oxidative stress in chronic exercise', *European Journal of Applied Physiology*, 111 (4), 695–705.

15 Yavari, A., Javadi, M., Mirmiran, P., and Bahadoran, Z. (2015), 'Exercise-induced oxidative stress and dietary antioxidants', *Asian Journal of Sports Medicine*, 6 (1), E24898.

16 Jamurtas, A. Z. (2018), 'Exercise-induced muscle damage and oxidative stress', *Antioxidants* (Basel, Switzerland), 7 (4), 50, https://doi.org/10.3390/antiox7040050.

17 Harty, P. S., Cottet, M. L., Malloy, J. K., and Kerksick, C. M. (2019), 'Nutritional and supplementation strategies to prevent and attenuate exercise-induced muscle damage: a brief review', *Sports Medicine – Open*, 5 (1), 1.

18 Huang, S., Rutkowsky, J., Snodgrass, R., Ono-Moore, K., et al. (2012), 'Saturated fatty acids activate TLR-mediated proinflammatory signaling pathways', *Journal of Lipid Research*, 53 (9), 2002–13.

19 Muñoz, A., and Costa, M. (2013), 'Nutritionally mediated oxidative stress and inflammation', *Oxidative Medicine and Cell Longevity*, 12, 610950.

20 Yuan, X. M., Anders, W. L., Olsson, A. G., Brunk, U. T. (1996), 'Iron in human atheroma and LDL oxidation by macrophages following erythrophagocytosis', *Atherosclerosis*, 124, 61–73.

21 Harasym, J., and Oledzki, R., 'Effect of fruit and vegetable antioxidants on total antioxidant capacity of blood plasma' (2014), *Nutrition*, 30 (5), 511–17.

22 Cömert, E., Mogol, B., and Gökmen, V. (2020), 'Relationship between color and antioxidant capacity of fruits and vegetables', *Current Research in Food Science*, 2, 1–10.

23 Shoba, G., Joy, D., Joseph, T., Majeed, M., Rajendran, R., and Srinivas, P. S. (1998), 'Influence of piperine on the pharmacokinetics of curcumin in animals and human volunteers', *Planta Medica*, 64 (4), 353–6.

24 NHS: The Eatwell Guide, https://www.nhs.uk/live-well/eat-well/the-eatwell-guide/.

25 Young, V. R., and Pellett, P. L. (1994), 'Plant proteins in relation to human protein and amino acid nutrition', *American Journal of Clinical Nutrition*, 59 (5 Suppl), 1203S–1212S.

26 Melina, V., Craig, W., and Levin, S. (2016), 'Position of the Academy of Nutrition and Dietetics: Vegetarian Diets', *Journal of the Academy of Nutrition and Dietetics*, 116 (12), 1970–80.

27 Seim, I., Ma, S., and Gladyshev, V. N. (2016), 'Gene expression signatures of human cell and tissue longevity', *NPJ Aging and Mechanisms of Disease*, 2, 16014, https://doi.org/10.1038/npjamd.

28 Sobiecki, J., Appleby, P., Bradbury, K., and Key, T. (2016), 'High compliance with dietary recommendations in a cohort of meat eaters, fish eaters, vegetarians, and

vegans: Results from the European Prospective Investigation into Cancer and Nutrition–Oxford study', *Nutrition Research*, 36 (5), 464–77.

29 Allès, B., Baudry, J., Méjean, C., Touvier, M., Péneau, S., Hercberg, S., Kesse-Guyot, E. (2017), 'Comparison of sociodemographic and nutritional characteristics between self-reported vegetarians, vegans, and meat-eaters from the NutriNet-Santé Study', *Nutrients*, 9 (9), ii, E1023.

30 Rizzo, N., Jaceldo-Siegl, K., Sabate, J., and Fraser, G. (2013), 'Nutrient profiles of vegetarian and nonvegetarian dietary patterns', *Journal of the Academy of Nutrition and Dietetics*, 113 (12), 1610–19.

31 Clarys, P., Deliens, T., Huybrechts, I., Deriemaeker, P., Vanaelst, B., De Keyzer, W., Hebbelinck, M., and Mullie, P. (2014), 'Comparison of nutritional quality of the vegan, vegetarian, semi-vegetarian, pesco-vegetarian and omnivorous diet', *Nutrient*, 6, 1318–32.

32 Kristensen, N. B., Madsen, M. L., Hansen, T. H., Allin, K. H., Hoppe, C., Fagt, S., Lausten, M. S., Gobel, R. J., Vestergaard, H., Hansen, T., et al. (2015), 'Intake of macro- and micronutrients in Danish vegans', *Nutrition Journal*, 14, 115.

33 Knuiman, P., Hopman, M. T. E., and Mensink, M., 'Glycogen availability and skeletal muscle adaptations with endurance and resistance exercise' (2015), *Nutrition and Metabolism* (Lond), 12, 59.

34 Phillips, S., Tipton, K., Aarsland, A., Wolf, S., and Wolfe, R. (1997), 'Mixed muscle protein synthesis and breakdown after resistance exercise in humans', *American Journal of Physiology*, 36 (1), E99–E107.

35 MacDougall, J. D., Gibala, M. J., Tarnopolsky, M. A., MacDonald, J. R., Interisano, S. A. and Yarasheski, K. E. (1995), 'The time course for elevated muscle protein synthesis following heavy resistance exercise', *Canadian Journal of Applied Physiology*, 20 (4), 480–86.

36 Tarnopolsky, M., Atkinson, S., Macdougall, J., Chesley, A., Phillips, S., and Schwarcz, H. (1992), 'Evaluation of protein requirements for trained strength athletes', *Journal of Applied Physiology*, 73 (5), 1986–95.

37 Morton, R., Murphy, K., McKellar, S., Schoenfeld, B., Henselmans, M., et al. (2018), 'A systematic review, meta-analysis and meta-regression of the effect of protein supplementation on resistance training-induced gains in muscle mass and strength in healthy adults', *British Journal of Sports Medicine*, 52 (6), 376–84.

38 Thomas, D. T., et al. (2016), 'Position of the Academy of Nutrition and Dietetics, Dietitians of Canada, and the American College of Sports Medicine: Nutrition and Athletic Performance', *Journal of the Academy of Nutrition and Dietetics*, 116, 3, 501–28.

39 Schoenfeld, B., Aragon, A., and Krieger, J. (2013), 'The effect of protein timing on muscle strength and hypertrophy: a meta-analysis', *Journal of the International Society of Sports Nutrition*, 10 (1), 53.

40 Wirth, J., Hillesheim, E., and Brennan, L. (2020), 'The role of protein intake and its timing on body composition and muscle function in healthy adults: a systematic review and meta-analysis of randomized controlled trials' (2020), *Journal of Nutrition*, 31 March.

41 Morton et al. (2018), op. cit.

42 Mamerow, M., Mettler, J., English, K., Casperson, S., et al. (2014), 'Dietary protein distribution positively influences 24-h muscle protein synthesis in healthy adults', *Journal of Nutrition*, 144 (6), 876-80.

43 Moore, D. R., Robinson, M. J., Fry, J. L., et al. (2009), 'Ingested protein dose response of muscle and albumin protein synthesis after resistance exercise in young men', *American Journal of Clinical Nutrition*, 89, 161–8.

44 Res, P. T., Groen, B., Pennings, B., Beelen, M., Wallis, G. A., Gijsen, A. P., Senden, J. M. G., and Van Loon, L. J. C. (2012), 'Protein Ingestion before Sleep Improves Postexercise Overnight Recovery', *Medicine & Science in Sports & Exercise*, 44 (8), 1560–69.

45 Snijders, T., Res, P., Smeets, J., Van Vliet, S., Van Kranenburg, J., et al. (2015), 'Protein ingestion before sleep increases muscle mass and strength gains during prolonged resistance-type exercise training in healthy young men 1-3', *Journal of Nutrition*, 145 (6), 1178–84A.

46 Mariotti F., 'Plant protein, animal protein, and protein quality', in: Mariotti, F. (ed.) (2017), *Vegetarian and Plant-Based Diets in Health and Disease Prevention*, Academic Press, Cambridge, MA, USA, 621–42.

47 Tomé, D. (2013), 'Digestibility issues of vegetable versus animal proteins: protein and amino acid requirements—functional aspects', *Food and Nutrition Bulletin*, 34 (2), 272–4.

48 Rand, W. M., Pellett, P. L., and Young, V. R. (2003), 'Meta-analysis of nitrogen balance studies for estimating protein requirements in healthy adults', *American Journal of Clinical Nutrition*, 77, 1, 109–27.

49 Abdulla, H., Smith, K., Atherton, P., and Idris, J. (2016), 'Role of insulin in the regulation of human skeletal muscle protein synthesis and breakdown: a systematic review and meta-analysis', *Diabetologia*, 59 (1), 44–55.

50 Greenhaff, P., Karagounis, L., Peirce, N., Simpson, E., Hazell, M., et al. (2008), 'Disassociation between the effects of amino acids and insulin on signaling, ubiquitin ligases, and protein turnover in human muscle', *American Journal of Physiology – Endocrinology and Metabolism*, 295 (3), E595–E604.

51 Bell, R., Al-Khalaf, M., and Megeney, L. (2016), 'The beneficial role of proteolysis in skeletal muscle growth and stress adaptation', *Skeletal Muscle*, 6 (16), 16.

Chapter 7: Performance

1 Fisher, I. (1908), *The Influence of Flesh-eating on Endurance*, Battle Creek, Mich., Modern Medicine Publishing.

2 Berry, E., 'The effects of a high and low protein diet on physical efficiency' (1909), *American Physical Education Review*, 14, 288–97.

3 Lynch, H. M., Wharton, C. M., and Johnston, C. S. (2016), 'Cardiorespiratory fitness and peak torque differences between vegetarian and omnivore endurance athletes: a cross-sectional study', *Nutrients*, 8 (11), 726.

4 Craddock, J., Probst, Y., and Peoples, G. (2016), 'Vegetarian and omnivorous nutrition – comparing physical performance', *International Journal of Sport Nutrition and Exercise Metabolism*, 26 (3), 212–20.

5 Yavari, A., Javadi, M., Mirmiran, P., and Bahadoran, Z. (2015), 'Exercise-induced oxidative stress and dietary antioxidants', *Asian Journal of Sports Medicine*, 6 (1), E24898.

6 Bondonno, C. P., Yang, X., Croft, K. D., Considine, M. J., Ward, N. C., Rich, L., Puddey, I. B., Swinny, E., Mubarak, A., and Hodgson, J. M. (2012), 'Flavonoid-rich apples and nitrate-rich spinach augment nitric oxide status and improve endothelial function in healthy men and women: a randomized controlled trial', *Free Radical Biology & Medicine*, 52 (1), 95–102.

7   Berry, N. M., Davison, K., Coates, A. M., Buckley, J. D., and Howe, P. R. (2010), 'Impact of cocoa flavanol consumption on blood pressure responsiveness to exercise', *British Journal of Nutrition*, 103 (10), 1480–84.

8   Richards, J. C., Lonac, M. C., Johnson, T. K., Schweder, M. M., and Bell, C. (2010), 'Epigallocatechin-3-gallate increases maximal oxygen uptake in adult humans', *Medicine & Science in Sports & Exercise*, 42 (4), 739–44.

9   Al-Dashti, Y., Holt, R., Stebbins, C., Keen, C., and Hackman, R. (2018), 'Dietary flavanols: a review of select effects on vascular function, blood pressure, and exercise performance', *Journal of the American College of Nutrition*, 37, 1–15.

10 ibid.

11 Ernst, E., and Franz, A., 'Blood fluidity score during vegetarian and hypocaloric diets – a pilot study' (1995), *Complementary Therapies in Medicine*, 3 (2), 70–71, doi: 10.1016/S0965-2299(95)80002-6.

12 Awodu, O., Makinde, Y. O., Adegbuyi, S. O., and Famodu, A. A. (2010), 'Short-term lacto-ovo-vegetarian diet and blood rheology in young Nigerian adults', *Annals of Biomedical Sciences*, 8, 10.4314/abs.v8i1.51716.

13 Ernst, E., Pietsch, L., Matrai, A., and Eisenberg, J. (1986), 'Blood rheology in vegetarians', *British Journal of Nutrition*, 56 (3), 555–60.

14 Naghedi-Baghdar, H., Nazari, S., Taghipour, A., Nematy, M., et al. (2018), 'Effect of diet on blood viscosity in healthy humans: a systematic review', *Electronic Physician*, 10 (3), 6563–70.

15 Ernst and Franz (1995), op. cit.

16 Smith, M., Lucas, A., Hamlin, R., and Devor, S. (2015), 'Associations among hemorheological factors and maximal oxygen consumption. Is there a role for blood viscosity in explaining athletic performance?', *Clinical Hemorheology and Microcirculation*, 60 (4), 347–62.

17 Nyberg, M., Gliemann, L., and Hellsten, Y. (2015), 'Vascular function in health, hypertension, and diabetes: effect of physical activity on skeletal muscle microcirculation', *Scandinavian Journal of Medicine & Science in Sports*, 25 (S4), 60–73.

18 Poole, D., Behnke, B., and Musch, T. (2020), 'The role of vascular function on exercise capacity in health and disease', *Journal of Physiology*, 24 January.

19 Domínguez, R., Cuenca, E., Maté-Muñoz, J. L., et al. (2017), 'Effects of beetroot juice supplementation on cardiorespiratory endurance in athletes, a systematic review', *Nutrients*, 9 (1), 43.

20 Hord, N. G., Tang, Y., and Bryan, N. S. (2009), 'Food sources of nitrates and nitrites: the physiologic context for potential health benefits', *American Journal of Clinical Nutrition*, 90, 1, 1–10.

21 Cantwell M., Elliott, C. (2017), 'Nitrates, nitrites and nitrosamines from processed meat intake and colorectal cancer risk', *Journal of Clinical Nutrition and Dietetics*, 3, 27.

22 Bartsch, H., Pignatelli, B., Calmels, S., and Ohshima, H. (1993), 'Inhibition of nitrosation', *Basic Life Sciences*, 61, 27–44.

23 Thomas, D. T., Erdman, K. A., and Burke, L. M. (2016), 'American College of Sports Medicine Joint Position Statement. Nutrition and athletic performance', *Medicine & Science in Sports & Exercise*, 48 (3), 543–68.

24 Hawley, J., and Leckey, A. (2015), 'Carbohydrate dependence during prolonged, intense endurance exercise', *Sports Medicine*, 45 (Suppl 1), 5–12.

25 Williams, C., and Rollo, I. (2015), 'Carbohydrate nutrition and team sport performance', *Sports Medicine*, 45 (Suppl 1), 13–22.

26 Couto, P., Bertuzzi, R., De Souza, C., Lima, H., Kiss, M., De-Oliveira, F., and Lima-Silva, A. (2015), 'High carbohydrate diet induces faster final sprint and overall 10,000-m times of young runners', *Pediatric Exercise Science*, 27 (3), 355–63.

27 Souglis, A., Chryssanthopoulos, C., Travlos, A., Zorzou, A., Gissis, I., Papadopoulos, C., and Sotiropoulos, A. (2012), 'The effect of high vs. low carbohydrate diets on distances covered in soccer', *Journal of Strength and Conditioning Research*/National Strength & Conditioning Association, 27.

28 Areta, J. L., Burke, L. M., Camera, D. M., et al. (2014), 'Reduced resting skeletal muscle protein synthesis is rescued by resistance exercise and protein ingestion following short-term energy deficit', *American Journal of Physiology–Endocrinology and Metabolism,* 306, E989–E997.

29 Rodriguez, N. R., Vislocky, L. M., and Gaine, P. C. (2007), 'Dietary protein, endurance exercise, and human skeletal-muscle protein turnover', *Current Opinion in Clinical Nutrition and Metabolic Care*, 10, 40–45.

30 Mettler, S., Mitchell, N., and Tipton, K. D. (2010), 'Increased protein intake reduces lean body mass loss during weight loss in athletes', *Medicine & Science in Sports & Exercise*, 42, 326–37.

31 Giles, G., Mahoney, C., Caruso, C., Bukhari, A., Smith, T., et al. (2019). 'Two days of calorie deprivation impairs high level cognitive processes, mood, and self-reported exertion during aerobic exercise: A randomized double-blind, placebo-controlled study', *Brain and Cognition*, 132, 33–40.

32 Subar, A., Kipnis, V., Troiano, R., Midthune, D., Schoeller, D., Bingham, S., and Schatzkin, A. (2003), 'Using intake biomarkers to evaluate the extent of dietary misreporting in a large sample of adults: the OPEN study', *American Journal of Epidemiology*, 158 (1), 1–13.

33 Champagne, C. M., Bray, G. A., Kurtz, A. A., Monteiro, J. B. R., Tucker, E., Volaufova, J., and Delany, J. P. (2002), 'Energy intake and energy expenditure: a controlled study comparing dietitians and non-dietitians', *Journal of the American Dietetic Association*, 102 (10), 1428–32.

34 Edmonds, C. J., Crombie, R., and Gardner, M. R, (2013), 'Subjective thirst moderates changes in speed of responding associated with water consumption', *Frontiers in Human Neuroscience*, 7, 363.

35 Rogers, P. J., Kainth, A., and Smit, H. J. (2001), 'A drink of water can improve or impair mental performance depending on small differences in thirst', *Appetite*, 36 (1), 57–8.

36 Neave, N., Scholey, A. B., Emmett, J. R., Moss, M., Kennedy, D. O., and Wesnes, K. A. (2001), 'Water ingestion improves subjective alertness, but has no effect on cognitive performance in dehydrated healthy young volunteers', *Appetite*, 37 (3), 255–6.

37 Bardis, C., Kavouras, S., Arnaoutis, G., Panagiotakos, D., and Sidossis, L. (2013), 'Mild dehydration and cycling performance during 5-kilometer hill climbing', *Journal of Athletic Training*, 48 (6), 741–7.

38 Jones, L. C., Cleary, M. A., Lopez, R. M., Zuri, R E., and Lopez, R. (2008), 'Active dehydration impairs upper and lower body anaerobic muscular power', *Journal of Strength and Conditioning Research*, 22 (2), 455–63.

39 American College of Sports Medicine, Sawka, M. N., Burke, L. M., Eichner, E. R., et al. (2007), 'American College of Sports Medicine position stand. Exercise and fluid replacement', *Medicine & Science in Sports & Exercise*, 39, 377–90.

40 ibid.

41 Burke, L. M., Kiens, B., and Ivy, J. L. (2004), 'Carbohydrates and fat for training and recovery', *Journal of Sports Sciences,* 22, 15–30.

42 Sherman, W. M., Brodowicz, D., Wright, D. A., Allen, W. K., Simonsen, J. and Dernbach, A. (1989), 'Effects of 4 h preexercise carbohydrate feedings on cycling performance', *Medicine & Science in Sports & Exercise,* 21 (5), 598–604.

43 Wright, D., Sherman, W., and Dernbach, A. (1991), 'Carbohydrate feedings before, during, or in combination improve cycling endurance performance', *Journal of Applied Physiology,* 71 (3), 1082–8.

44 Schabort, E. J., Bosch, A. N., Weltan, S. M., and Noakes, T. D. (1999), 'The effect of a preexercise meal on time to fatigue during prolonged cycling exercise', *Medicine & Science in Sports & Exercise,* 31 (3), 464–71.

45 Maffucci, D., and McMurray, R. (2000), 'Towards optimizing the timing of the pre-exercise meal', *International Journal of Sport Nutrition and Exercise Metabolism,* 10 (2), 103–13.

46. Ormsbee, M. J., Bach, C. W., and Baur, D. A. (2014), 'Pre-exercise nutrition: the role of macronutrients, modified starches and supplements on metabolism and endurance performance', *Nutrients,* 6, 1782–1808.

47 Rehrer, N. J., van Kemenade, M., Meester, W., Brouns, F., and Saris, W. H. (1992), 'Gastrointestinal complaints in relation to dietary intake in triathletes', *International Journal of Sport Nutrition,* 2, 48–59.

48 Wong, S., Sun, F., Yajun, C., Li, C., Zhang, Y., and Huang, W. Y. (2017), 'Effect of pre-exercise carbohydrate diets with high vs low glycemic index on exercise performance: a meta-analysis', *Nutrition Reviews,* 75, 10.1093/nutrit/nux003.

49 Kim, J. S., Nam, K., and Chung, S. J. (2019), 'Effect of nutrient composition in a mixed meal on the postprandial glycemic response in healthy people: a preliminary study', *Nutrition Research and Practice,* 13 (2), 126–33.

50 Wong, et al. (2017), op. cit.

51 Jeukendrup, A. E. (2013), 'Oral carbohydrate rinse: placebo or beneficial?', *Current Sports Medicine Reports,* 12 (4), 222–7.

52 Burke, L., and Maughan, R. (2015), 'The Governor has a sweet tooth – mouth sensing of nutrients to enhance sports performance', *European Journal of Sport Science:* Current Controversies in Sports Nutrition, 24 (4), 29–40.

53 Pöchmüller, M., Schwingshackl, L., Colombani, P. C., et al. (2016), 'A systematic review and meta-analysis of carbohydrate benefits associated with randomized controlled competition-based performance trials', *Journal of the International Society of Sports Nutrition,* 13, 27.

54 Jeukendrup, A. (2010), 'Carbohydrate and exercise performance: the role of multiple transportable carbohydrates', *Current Opinion in Clinical Nutrition and Metabolic Care,* 13, 452–7.

55 Canadian Sugar Institute: Sources of Sugar, https://sugar.ca/Sugar-Basics/Sources-of-Sugar.aspx.

56 Burke, L. M., Kiens, B., and Ivy, J. L. (2004), 'Carbohydrates and fat for training and recovery', *Journal of Sports Sciences,* 22, 15–30.

57 Hawley, J. A., Schabort, E. J., Noakes, T. D., and Dennis, S. C. (1997), 'Carbohydrate-loading and exercise performance. An update', *Sports Medicine,* 24, 73–81.

58 Burke, L., Hawley, J., Wong, S., and Jeukendrup, A. (2011), 'Carbohydrates for training and competition', *Journal of Sports Sciences,* 29, 17.

59 Bussau, V., Fairchild, A., Rao, T., Steele, J., and Fournier, A. (2002), 'Carbohydrate loading in human muscle: an improved 1 day protocol', *European Journal of Applied Physiology,* 87 (3), 290–95.

60 Australian Institute of Sport: The AIS Sports Supplement Framework, https://www.ais.gov.au/__data/assets/pdf_file/0004/698557/AIS-Sports-Supplement-Framework-2019.pdf.

61 Thomas, D. T., et al., 'American College of Sports Medicine Joint Position Statement'.

62 Reyes, C. M., and Cornelis, M. C. (2018), 'Caffeine in the Diet: Country-Level Consumption and Guidelines', *Nutrients*, 10 (11), 1772.

63 Grgic, J., Grgic, I., Pickering, C., et al. (2020), 'Wake up and smell the coffee: caffeine supplementation and exercise performance – an umbrella review of 21 published meta-analyses', *British Journal of Sports Medicine*, 54, 681–8.

64 Davis, J. K., Green, J. M. (2009), 'Caffeine and anaerobic performance: ergogenic value and mechanisms of action', *Sports Medicine*, 39, 813–32.

65 Fredholm, B. (1995), 'Adenosine, adenosine receptors and the actions of caffeine', *Pharmacology & Toxicology*, 76 (2), 93–101.

66 Zhang, Y., Coca, A., Casa, D., Antonio, J., Green, J., and Bishop, P. (2015), 'Caffeine and diuresis during rest and exercise: a meta-analysis', *Journal of Science and Medicine in Sport*, 18 (5), 569–74.

67 Gonçalves, L. S., Painelli, V. S., Yamaguchi, G., et al. (2017), 'Dispelling the myth that habitual caffeine consumption influences the performance response to acute caffeine supplementation', *Journal of Applied Physiology*, 123, 213–20.

68 Spriet, L. (2014), 'Exercise and sport performance with low doses of caffeine', *Sports Medicine*, 44 (Suppl 2), 175–84.

69 Balsom, P. D., Söderlund, K., and Ekblom, B. (1994), 'Creatine in humans with special reference to creatine supplementation', *Sports Medicine* (Auckland, NZ), 18 (4), 268–80.

70 Kreider, R. B., and Jung, Y. P. (2011), 'Creatine supplementation in exercise, sport, and medicine', *Journal of Exercise, Nutrition and Biochemistry*, 15 (2), 53–69.

71 ibid.

72 Lanhers, C., et al. (2015), 'Creatine supplementation and lower limb strength performance: a systematic review and meta-analyses', *Sports Medicine*, 45 (9), 1285–94.

73 Lanhers, C., Pereira, B., Naughton, G., Trousselard, M., Lesage, F. X., and Dutheil, F. (2016), 'Creatine supplementation and upper limb strength performance: a systematic review and meta-analysis', *Sports Medicine* (Auckland, NZ), 47, 10.1007/s40279-016-0571-4.

74 Mielgo-Ayuso, J., Calleja-Gonzalez, J., Marqués-Jiménez, D., Caballero-García, A., Córdova, A. and Fernández-Lázaro, D. (2019), 'Effects of creatine supplementation on athletic performance in soccer players: a systematic review and meta-analysis', *Nutrients*, 11 (4), 757.

75 Chilibeck, P. D., Kaviani, M., Candow, D. G., and Zello, G. A. (2017), 'Effect of creatine supplementation during resistance training on lean tissue mass and muscular strength in older adults: a meta-analysis', *Journal of Sports Medicine*, 8, 213–26.

76 Burke, D. G., Candow, D. G., Chilibeck, P. D., MacNeil, L. G., Roy, B. D., Tarnopolsky, M. A., and Ziegenfuss, T. (2008), 'Effect of creatine supplementation and resistance-exercise training on muscle insulin-like growth factor in young adults', *International Journal of Sport Nutrition and Exercise Metabolism*, 18, 389–98.

77 Burke, D., Chilibeck, P., Parise, G., Candow, D., Mahoney, D., and Tarnopolsky, M. (2003), 'Effect of creatine and weight training on muscle creatine and performance in vegetarians', *Medicine & Science in sports & exercise*, 35, 1946–55.

78 Buford, T. W., Kreider, R. B., Stout, J. R., et al. (2007), 'International Society of Sports Nutrition position stand: Creatine supplementation and exercise', *Journal of the International Society of Sports Nutrition*, 4, 6.

79 Forbes, S. C., and Candow, D. G. (2018), 'Timing of creatine supplementation and resistance training: a brief review', *Journal of Exercise and Nutrition*, 1 (5).

80 Candow, D. G., Vogt, E., Johannsmeyer, S., Forbes, S. C., and Farthing, J. P. (2015), 'Strategic creatine supplementation and resistance training in healthy older adults', *Applied Physiology, Nutrition, and Metabolism = Physiologie appliquée, nutrition et métabolisme*, 40 (7), 689–94.

81 Antonio, J., and Ciccone, V. (2013), 'The effects of pre versus post workout supplementation of creatine monohydrate on body composition and strength', *Journal of the International Society of Sports Nutrition*, 10, 36.

82 Cooper, R., Naclerio, F., Allgrove, J., and Jimenez, A. (2012), 'Creatine supplementation with specific view to exercise/sports performance: an update', *Journal of the International Society of Sports Nutrition*, 9 (1), 33, https://doi.org/10.1186/1550-2783-9-33.

83 Knapik, J. J., et al. (2016), 'Prevalence of dietary supplement use by athletes: systematic review and meta-analysis', *Sports Medicine*, 46 (1), 103–23.

84 Waddington, I., Malcolm, D., Roderick, M., Naik, R., and Spitzer, G. (2005), 'Drug use in English professional football', *British Journal of Sports Medicine*, 39 (4), E18; discussion e18.

85 Kreider, R. B., Kalman, D. S., Antonio, J., et al. (2017), 'International Society of Sports Nutrition position stand: safety and efficacy of creatine supplementation in exercise, sport, and medicine', *Journal of the International Society of Sports Nutrition*, 14, 18.

86 Kreider, R. B., et al. (2003), 'Long-term creatine supplementation does not significantly affect clinical markers of health in athletes', *Molecular and Cellular Biochemistry*, 244 (1–2), 95–104.

87 Greenwood, M., et al. (2003), 'Creatine supplementation during college football training does not increase the incidence of cramping or injury', *Molecular and Cellular Biochemistry*, 244 (1–2), 83–8.

88 Mielgo-Ayuso, et al. (2019), op. cit. 'Effects of creatine supplementation on athletic performance in soccer players'.

89 Maughan, R. (2018), 'Dietary supplements and the high-performance athlete', *International Journal of Sport Nutrition and Exercise Metabolism*, 28 (2), 101.

90 Jonvik, K., Nyakayiru, J., van Dijk, J., Wardenaar, F., van Loon, L., and Verdijk, L. (2016), 'Habitual dietary nitrate intake in highly trained athletes', *International Journal of Sport Nutrition and Exercise Metabolism*, 27, 1-25, 10.1123/ijsnem.2016-0239.

91 Linoby, A., et al. (2020), 'The role of fitness status in the performance-enhancing effects of dietary inorganic nitrate supplementation: meta-analysis and meta-regression analysis', in: Hassan, M., et al. (eds), *Enhancing Health and Sports Performance by Design*, MoHE 2019, Lecture Notes in Bioengineering, Springer, Singapore.

92 Flueck, J., Bogdanova, A., Mettler, S., and Perret, C. (2016), 'Is beetroot juice more effective than sodium nitrate? The effects of equimolar nitrate dosages of nitrate-rich beetroot juice and sodium nitrate on oxygen consumption during exercise', *Applied Physiology, Nutrition, and Metabolism*, 41 (4), 421–9.

93 Domínguez, R., Cuenca, E., Maté-Muñoz, J. L., García-Fernández, P., Serra-Paya, N., Estevan, M. C., Herreros, P. V., and Garnacho-Castaño, M. V. (2017), 'Effects of beetroot juice supplementation on cardiorespiratory endurance in athletes. A systematic review', *Nutrients*, 9 (1), 43.

94 Jones, A. M., 'Influence of dietary nitrate on the physiological determinants of exercise performance: A critical review 1.' (2014), *Applied Physiology, Nutrition, and Metabolism*, 39(9), 1019–1028.

95 Domínguez, R., Maté-Muñoz, J. L., Cuenca, E., et al. (2018), 'Effects of beetroot juice supplementation on intermittent high-intensity exercise efforts', *Journal of the International Society of Sports Nutrition,* 15, 2.

96 Larsen, F., Weitzberg, E., Lundberg, J., and Ekblom, B. (2007), 'Effects of dietary nitrate on oxygen cost during exercise', *Acta Physiologica,* 191 (1), 59–66.

97 Bailey, S., Winyard, P., Vanhatalo, A., Blackwell, J., DiMenna, F. J., et al. (2009), 'Dietary nitrate supplementation reduces the O2 cost of low-intensity exercise and enhances tolerance to high-intensity exercise in humans', *Journal of Applied Physiology,* 107 (4), 1144–55.

98 Domínguez et al. (2018), op. cit.

99 Lansley, K. E., Winyard, P. G., Fulford, J., Vanhatalo, A., Bailey, S. J., Blackwell, J. R., DiMenna, F. J., Gilchrist, M., Benjamin, N., and Jones, A. M. (2011), 'Dietary nitrate supplementation reduces the O2 cost of walking and running: a placebo-controlled study', *Journal of Applied Physiology,* 110 (3), 591–600.

100 Peeling, P., Cox, G. R., Bullock, N., and Burke, L. M. (2015), 'Beetroot juice improves on-water 500 M time-trial performance, and laboratory-based paddling economy in national and international-level kayak athletes', *International Journal of Sport Nutrition and Exercise Metabolism,* 25 (3), 278–84.

101 Thompson, C., Wylie, L. J., Fulford, J., Kelly, J., Black, M. I., McDonagh, S. T. J., et al. (2015), 'Dietary nitrate improves sprint performance and cognitive function during prolonged intermittent exercise', *European Journal of Applied Physiology,* 115, 1825–34.

102 Mosher, S. L., Sparks, S. A., Williams, E. J., Bentley, D. R., and McNaughton, L. (2016), 'Ingestion of a nitric oxide enhancing supplement improves resistance exercise performance', *Journal of Strength and Conditioning Research,* 30 (12), 3520–24.

103 Linoby et al. (2020), op. cit.

104 Domínguez et al. (2018), op. cit.

105 Gallardo, E. J., and Coggan, A. R. (2019), 'What's in your beet juice? Nitrate and nitrite content of beet juice products marketed to athletes', *International Journal of Sport Nutrition and Exercise Metabolism,* 29 (4), 345–9.

106 Peeling et al. (2015), op. cit.

107 Bryan, N., Alexander, D., Coughlin, J., Milkowski, A., and Boffetta, P. (2012), 'Ingested nitrate and nitrite and stomach cancer risk: an updated review', *Food and Chemical Toxicology,* 50 (10), 3646–65.

108 Hobson, R., Saunders, M., Ball, B., Harris, G., and Sale, C. (2012), 'Effects of β-alanine supplementation on exercise performance: A meta-analysis', *Amino Acids,* 43 (1), 25–37.

109 Saunders, B., Elliott-Sale, K., Artioli, G., Swinton, P., et al. (2017), 'β-alanine supplementation to improve exercise capacity and performance: a systematic review and meta-analysis', *British Journal of Sports Medicine,* 51 (8), 658–69.

110 Everaert, I., Mooyaart, A., Baguet, A., Zutinic, et al. (2011), 'Vegetarianism, female gender and increasing age, but not CNDP1 genotype, are associated with reduced muscle carnosine levels in humans', *Amino Acids,* 40 (4), 1221–9.

111 Harris, R. C., Wise, J. A., Price, K. A., Kim, H. J., Kim, C. K., and Sale, C. (2012), 'Determinants of muscle carnosine content', *Amino Acids,* 43 (1), 5–12.

112 Rogerson, D. (2017), 'Vegan diets: practical advice for athletes and exercisers', *Journal of the International Society of Sports Nutrition,* 14, 36.

113 Peeling, P., Binnie, M., Goods, P., Sim, M., and Burke, L. (2018), 'Evidence-based supplements for the enhancement of athletic performance', *International Journal of Sport Nutrition and Exercise Metabolism,* 28 (2), 178–87.

114 Chung, W., Shaw, G., Anderson, M. E., Pyne, D. B., Saunders, P. U., Bishop, D. J., and Burke, L. M. (2012), 'Effect of 10 week beta-alanine supplementation on competition and training performance in elite swimmers', *Nutrients*, 4 (12), 1441–53.

115 Baguet, A., Bourgois, J., Vanhee, L., Achten, E., and Derave, W. (2010), 'Important role of muscle carnosine in rowing performance', *Journal of Applied Physiology* (1985), 109 (4), 1096–1101.

116 Carr, A. J., Hopkins, W. G., and Gore, C. J. (2011), 'Effects of acute alkalosis and acidosis on performance: a meta-analysis', *Sports Medicine*, 41 (10), 801–14.

117 Lancha Junior, A. H., de Painelli, V. S., Saunders, B., and Artioli, G. G. (2015), 'Nutritional strategies to modulate intracellular and extracellular buffering capacity during high-intensity exercise', *Sports Medicine*, 45 (Suppl. 1), 71–81.

118 Carr, A. J., Slater, G. J., Gore, C. J., Dawson, B., and Burke, L. M. (2011), 'Effect of sodium bicarbonate on [HCO_3 −], pH, and gastrointestinal symptoms', *International Journal of Sport Nutrition and Exercise Metabolism*, 21 (3), 189–94.

119 Krustrup, P., Ermidis, G., and Mohr, M. (2015), 'Sodium bicarbonate intake improves high-intensity intermittent exercise performance in trained young men', *Journal of the International Society of Sports Nutrition*, 12, 25.

Chapter 8: Other important lifestyle habits for health and performance

1 YouGov: Three Quarters Brits Get Less Than Eight Hours Sleep, https://yougov.co.uk/topics/health/articles-reports/2020/01/17/three-quarters-brits-get-less-eight-hours-sleep.

2 Lo, K., Woo, B., Wong, M., and Tam, W. (2018), 'Subjective sleep quality, blood pressure, and hypertension: a meta-analysis', *Journal of Clinical Hypertension* (Greenwich, Conn.), 20 (3), 592–605.

3 Wang, Y., Mei, H., Jiang, Y.-R., Sun, W.-Q., Song, Y.-J., Liu, S.-J., and Jiang, F. (2015), 'Relationship between duration of sleep and hypertension in adults: a meta-analysis', *Journal of Clinical Sleep Medicine*, 11 (9), 1047–56.

4 Krittanawong, C., Tunhasiriwet, A., Wang, Z., Zhang, H., et al. (2017), 'Association between short and long sleep duration and cardiovascular outcomes? A systematic review and meta-analysis', *Journal of the American College of Cardiology*, 69 (11), 1798.

5 Bubu, O., Brannick, M., Mortimer, J., Umasabor-Bubu, O., et al. (2017), 'Sleep, cognitive impairment, and Alzheimer's disease: a systematic review and meta-analysis', *Sleep*, 40 (1).

6 Shan, Z., Ma, H., Xie, M., Yan, P., et al. (2015), 'Sleep duration and risk of type 2 diabetes: a meta-analysis of prospective studies', *Diabetes Care, 38* (3), 529–37.

7 Wu, Y., Zhai, L., and Zhang, D. (2014), 'Sleep duration and obesity among adults: a meta-analysis of prospective studies', *Sleep Medicine,* 92 (1), 111–20.

8 Fatima, Y., Doi, S., and Mamun, A. (2016), 'Sleep quality and obesity in young subjects: a meta-analysis', *Obesity Reviews*, 17 (11), 1154–66.

9 Stenholm, S., Head, J., Kivimäki, M., Magnusson Hanson, L. L., et al. (2019), 'Sleep duration and sleep disturbances as predictors of healthy and chronic disease-free life expectancy between ages 50 and 75: a pooled analysis of three cohorts', *Journals of Gerontology Series A: Biomedical Sciences and Medical Sciences*, 74 (2), 204–10.

10 Cappuccio, F. P., D'Elia, L., Strazzullo, P., and Miller, M. A. (2010), 'Sleep duration and all-cause mortality: a systematic review and meta-analysis of prospective studies', *Sleep, 33* (5), 585–92, https://doi.org/10.1093/sleep/33.5.585.

11 Irwin, M., Olmstead, R., and Carroll, J. (2016), 'Sleep disturbance, sleep duration, and inflammation: a systematic review and meta-analysis of cohort studies and experimental sleep deprivation', *Biological Psychiatry*, 80 (1), 40–52.

12 Wu, Y., Zhai, L., and Zhang, D. (2014), 'Sleep duration and obesity among adults: a meta-analysis of prospective studies', *Sleep Medicine*, 92 (1), 111–20.

13 Zhou, Q., Zhang, M., and Hu, D. (2019), 'Dose-response association between sleep duration and obesity risk: a systematic review and meta-analysis of prospective cohort studies', *Sleep and Breathing*, 23 (4), 1035–45.

14 Sperry, S., Scully, I., Gramzow, R., and Jorgensen, R. (2015), 'Sleep duration and waist circumference in adults: a meta-analysis', *Sleep*, 38 (8), 1269–76.

15 Spiegel, K., Tasali, E., Penev, P., and Van Cauter, E. (2004), 'Brief communication: sleep curtailment in healthy young men is associated with decreased leptin levels, elevated ghrelin levels, and increased hunger and appetite', *Annals of Internal Medicine*, 141 (11), 846–50.

16 Spiegel, K., Leproult, R., L'Hermite-Balériaux, M., Copinschi, G., Penev, P., and Van Cauter, E. (2004), 'Leptin levels are dependent on sleep duration: relationships with sympathovagal balance, carbohydrate regulation, cortisol, and thyrotropin', *Journal of Clinical Endocrinology and Metabolism*, 89(11), 5762–71.

17 St-Onge, M.-P., Wolfe, S., Sy, M., Shechter, A., and Hirsch, J. (2013), 'Sleep restriction increases the neuronal response to unhealthy food in normal-weight individuals', *International Journal of Obesity*, 38 (3), 411–16.

18 Zhai, L., Zhang, H., and Zhang, D. (2015), 'Sleep duration and depression among adults: a meta-analysis of prospective studies', *Depression and Anxiety*, 32 (9), 664–70.

19 Cox, R., and Olatunji, B. (2020), 'Sleep in the anxiety-related disorders: a meta-analysis of subjective and objective research', *Sleep Medicine Reviews*, 51, 101282.

20 Alvaro, P., Roberts, R., and Harris, J. (2013), 'A systematic review assessing bidirectionality between sleep disturbances, anxiety, and depression', *Sleep*, 36 (7), 1059–68.

21 Steptoe, A., O'Donnell, K., Marmot, M., and Wardle, J. (2008), 'Positive affect, psychological well-being, and good sleep', *Journal of Psychosomatic Research*, 64 (4), 409–15.

22 Ong, A., Exner-Cortens, D., Riffin, D., Steptoe, C., Zautra, A., and Almeida, A. (2013), 'Linking stable and dynamic features of positive affect to sleep', *Annals of Behavioral Medicine*, 46 (1), 52–61.

23 Lastella, M., Roach, G., Halson, S., and Sargent, C. (2015), 'Sleep/wake behaviours of elite athletes from individual and team sports', *European Journal of Sport Science*, 15 (2), 94–100.

24 Vlahoyiannis, A., Aphamis, G., Bogdanis, G., Sakkas, G., Andreou, E., and Giannaki, C. (2020), 'Deconstructing athletes' sleep: a systematic review of the influence of age, sex, athletic expertise, sport type, and season on sleep characteristics', *Journal of Sport and Health Science*, 1–17.

25 Roberts, S., Teo, W., and Warmington, S. (2019), 'Effects of training and competition on the sleep of elite athletes: a systematic review and meta-analysis', *British Journal of Sports Medicine*, 53 (8), 513–22.

26 Lim, J., and Dinges, D. (2010), 'A meta-analysis of the impact of short-term sleep deprivation on cognitive variables', *Psychological Bulletin*, 136 (3), 375–89.

27 Rasch, B., and Born, J. (2013), 'About sleep's role in memory', *Physiological Reviews*, 93, 681–766.

28 Leong, R., Cheng, G., Chee, M., and Lo, J. (2019), 'The effects of sleep on prospective memory: a systematic review and meta-analysis', *Sleep Medicine Reviews*, 47, 18–27.

29 Reyner, L. A., Horne, J. A. (2013), 'Sleep restriction and serving accuracy in performance tennis players, and effects of caffeine', *Physiology and Behavior*, 120, 93–6.

30 Mah, C. D., Mah, K. E., Kezirian, E. J., and Dement, W. C. (2011), 'The effects of sleep extension on the athletic performance of collegiate basketball players', *Sleep*, 34 (7), 943–50, https://doi.org/10.5665/SLEEP.1132.

31 Pallesen, S., Gundersen, H., Kristoffersen, M., Bjorvatn, B., Thun, E., and Harris, A. (2017), 'The effects of sleep deprivation on soccer skills', *Perceptual and Motor Skills*, 124 (4), 812–29.

32 Oliver, S., Costa, J., Laing, R., Bilzon, S., and Walsh, S. (2009), 'One night of sleep deprivation decreases treadmill endurance performance', *European Journal of Applied Physiology*, 107 (2), 155–61.

33 Roberts, S., Teo, W. P., Aisbett, B., and Warmington, S. A. (2019), 'Extended sleep maintains endurance performance better than normal or restricted sleep', *Medicine and Science in Sports and Exercise*, 51 (12), 2516–23.

34 Bonnar, D., Bartel, K., Kakoschke, N., & Lang, C. (2018), 'Sleep interventions designed to improve athletic performance and recovery: a systematic review of current approaches', *Sports Medicine* (Auckland, NZ), 48 (3), 683–703.

35 Fullagar, H., Skorski, H., Duffield, K., Hammes, S., Coutts, R., and Meyer, D. (2015), 'Sleep and athletic performance: the effects of sleep loss on exercise performance, and physiological and cognitive responses to exercise', *Sports Medicine*, 45 (2), 161–86.

36 Skein, M. J., Duffield, R., Edge, J., Short, M., and Mündel, T. (2011), 'Intermittent-sprint performance and muscle glycogen after 30 h of sleep deprivation', *Medicine & Science in Sports & Exercise*, 43 (7), 1301–11.

37 Lamon, S., Morabito, A., Arentson-Lantz, E., Knowles, O., et al. (2020), 'The effect of acute sleep deprivation on skeletal muscle protein synthesis and the hormonal environment', *BioRxiv*, 11 March.

38 Aisbett, B., Condo, D., Zacharewicz, E., and Lamon, S. (2017), 'The impact of shift-work on skeletal muscle health', *Nutrients*, 9 (3), 248.

39 Milewski, M. D., Skaggs, D. L., Bishop, G. A., Pace, J. L., Ibrahim, D. A., Wren, T. A. L., and Barzdukas, A. (2014), 'Chronic lack of sleep is associated with increased sports injuries in adolescent athletes', *Journal of Pediatric Orthopaedics*, 34 (2), 129–33.

40 Von Rosen, P., Frohm, A., Kottorp, A., Fridén, C., and Heijne, A. (2017), 'Multiple factors explain injury risk in adolescent elite athletes: applying a biopsychosocial perspective', *Scandinavian Journal of Medicine & Science in Sports*, 27 (12), 2059–69.

41 Cohen, S., Doyle, W., Alper, C., Janicki-Deverts, D., and Turner, R. (2009), 'Sleep habits and susceptibility to the common cold', *Archives of Internal Medicine*, 169 (1), 62–7.

42 Prather, A., Janicki-Deverts, D., Hall, M., and Cohen, S. (2015), 'Behaviorally assessed sleep and susceptibility to the common cold', *Sleep*, 38 (9), 1353–9.

43 Súdy, A. R., Ella, K., Bódizs, R., and Káldi, K. (2019), 'Association of social jetlag with sleep quality and autonomic cardiac control during sleep in young healthy men', *Frontiers in Neuroscience*, 13, 950.

44 Ebrahim, I. O., Shapiro, C. M., Williams, A. J., and Fenwick, P. B. (2013), 'Alcohol and sleep I: effects on normal sleep', *Alcoholism, Clinical and Experimental Research*, 37 (4), 539–49.

45 Simon, J., and Docherty, C. (2017), 'The impact of previous athletic experience on current physical fitness in former collegiate athletes and noncollegiate athletes', *Sports Health: A Multidisciplinary Approach*, 9 (5), 462–8.

46 Strawbridge, M. (2001), 'Current activity patterns of women intercollegiate athletes of the late 1960's and 1970's', *Women in Sport & Physical Activity Journal*, 10 (1), 55.

47 Cheng, W., Zhang, Z., Cheng, W., Yang, C., Diao, L., and Liu, W. (2018), 'Associations of leisure-time physical activity with cardiovascular mortality: a systematic review and meta-analysis of 44 prospective cohort studies', *European Journal of Preventive Cardiology*, 25 (17), 1864–72.

48 Aune, D., Norat, T., Leitzmann, M., Tonstad, S., and Vatten, L. J. (2015), 'Physical activity and the risk of type 2 diabetes: a systematic review and dose-response meta-analysis', *European Journal of Epidemiology*, 30 (7), 529–42.

49 Zhong, S., Ma, T., Chen, L., Chen, W., Lv, M., Zhang, X., and Zhao, J. (2016), 'Physical activity and risk of lung cancer: a meta-analysis', *Clinical Journal of Sport Medicine*, 26 (3), 173–81.

50 Kyu, H., Bachman, V., Alexander, L., Mumford, J., et al. (2016), 'Physical activity and risk of breast cancer, colon cancer, diabetes, ischemic heart disease, and ischemic stroke events: systematic review and dose-response meta-analysis for the Global Burden of Disease Study 2013', *British Medical Journal*, 354, I3857.

51 Kim, H., Reece, J., and Kang, M. (2020), 'Effects of accumulated short bouts of exercise on weight and obesity indices in adults: a meta-analysis', *American Journal of Health Promotion*, 34 (1), 96–104.

52 Guure, C., Ibrahim, N., Adam, M., and Said, S. (2017), 'Impact of physical activity on cognitive decline, dementia, and its subtypes: meta-analysis of prospective studies', *BioMed Research International*, 13.

53 Blond, K., Brinkløv, C. F., Ried-Larsen, M., Crippa, A., and Grøntved, A. (2019), 'Association of high amounts of physical activity with mortality risk: a systematic review and meta-analysis, *British Journal of Sports Medicine*, Bjsports-2018-100393.

54 Mist, S. D., Firestone, K. A., and Jones, K. D. (2013), 'Complementary and alternative exercise for fibromyalgia: a meta-analysis', *Journal of Pain Research*, 6, 247–60.

55 Hong, A. R., and Kim, S. W. (2018), 'Effects of resistance exercise on bone health', *Endocrinology and metabolism* (Seoul, Korea), 33 (4), 435–44.

56 de Mello, R., Dalla Corte, R. R., Gioscia, J., and Moriguchi, E. H. (2019), 'Effects of physical exercise programs on sarcopenia management, dynapenia, and physical performance in the elderly: a systematic review of randomized clinical trials' (2019), *Journal of Aging Research*, 1959486.

57 Mcdowell, C., Dishman, R., Gordon, B., and Herring, M. (2019), 'Physical activity and anxiety: a systematic review and meta-analysis of prospective cohort studies', *American Journal of Preventive Medicine*, 57 (4), 545–56.

58 Schuch, F., Vancampfort, D., Firth, J., Rosenbaum, et al. (2018), 'Physical activity and incident depression: a meta-analysis of prospective cohort studies', *American Journal of Psychiatry*, 175 (7), 631–48.

59 Aylett, E., Small, N., and Bower, P. (2018), 'Exercise in the treatment of clinical anxiety in general practice – a systematic review and meta-analysis', *BMC Health Services Research*, 18 (1), 559.

60 Schuch, F., Vancampfort, D., Richards, J., Rosenbaum, S., Ward, P., and Stubbs, B. (2016), 'Exercise as a treatment for depression: a meta-analysis adjusting for publication bias', *Journal of Psychiatric Research*, 77, 42–51.

61 Thompson Coon, J., Boddy, K., Stein, K., Whear, R., Barton, J., and Depledge, M. H. (2011), 'Does participating in physical activity in outdoor natural environments have a greater effect on physical and mental wellbeing than physical activity indoors? A systematic review', *Environmental Science & Technology*, 45 (5), 1761–72.

62 Zhang, Z., and Chen, W. (2019), 'A systematic review of the relationship between physical activity and happiness', *Journal of Happiness Studies*, 20 (4), 1305–22.

63 Puetz, T. W. (2006), 'Physical activity and feelings of energy and fatigue: epidemiological evidence', *Sports Medicine* (Auckland, NZ), 36 (9), 767–80.

64 Eime, R. M., Young, J. A., Harvey, J. T., Charity, M. J., and Payne, W. R. (2013), 'A systematic review of the psychological and social benefits of participation in sport for adults: informing development of a conceptual model of health through sport', *International Journal of Behavioral Nutrition and Physical Activity*, 10, 135.

65 Stanton, A., Handy, A., and Meston, C. (2018), 'The effects of exercise on sexual function in women', *Sexual Medicine Reviews*, 6 (4), 548–57.

66 Silva, A. B., Sousa, N., Azevedo, L. F., and Martins, C. (2017), 'Physical activity and exercise for erectile dysfunction: systematic review and meta-analysis', *British Journal of Sports Medicine*, 51 (19), 1419–24.

67 D'Andrea, S., Spaggiari, G., Barbonetti, A., et al. (2020), 'Endogenous transient doping: physical exercise acutely increases testosterone levels—results from a meta-analysis', *Journal of Endocrinological Investigation*, 10.1007/s40618-020-01251-3. Advance online publication.

68 Anderson, R. M. (2013), 'Positive sexuality and its impact on overall well-being', *Bundesgesundheitsblatt Gesundheitsforschung Gesundheitsschutz*, 56 (2), 208–14.

69 Kelley, G. A., and Kelley, K. S. (2017), 'Exercise and sleep: a systematic review of previous meta-analyses', *Journal of Evidence-based Medicine*, 10 (1), 26–36.

70 Chau, J., Grunseit, A., Chey, T., Stamatakis, E., et al. (2013), 'Daily sitting time and all-cause mortality: a meta-analysis', *PLoS ONE*, 8 (11), E80000.

71 Parsons, T. J., Sartini, C. T., Welsh, P. G., Sattar, N. H., et al. (2017), 'Physical activity, sedentary behavior, and inflammatory and hemostatic markers in men', *Medicine & Science in Sports & Exercise*, 49 (3), 459–65.

72 Eddy, P., Heckenberg, R., Wertheim, E., Kent, S., and Wright, B. (2016), 'A systematic review and meta-analysis of the effort–reward imbalance model of workplace stress with indicators of immune function', *Journal of Psychosomatic Research*, 91, 1.

73 Konturek, P. C., Brzozowski, T., and Konturek, S. J. (2011), 'Stress and the gut: pathophysiology, clinical consequences, diagnostic approach and treatment options', *Journal of Physiology and Pharmacology*, 62 (6), 591–9.

74 Booth, J., Connelly, L., Lawrence, M., Chalmers, C., Joice, S., Becker, C., and Dougall, N. (2015), 'Evidence of perceived psychosocial stress as a risk factor for stroke in adults: a meta-analysis', *BMC Neurology*, 15, 233.

75 Richardson, S., Shaffer, J. A., Falzon, L., Krupka, D., Davidson, K. W., and Edmondson, D. (2012), 'Meta-analysis of perceived stress and its association with incident coronary heart disease', *American Journal of Cardiology*, 110 (12), 1711–16.

76 French, K., Allen, T., and Henderson, T. (2019), 'Challenge and hindrance stressors in relation to sleep', *Social Science & Medicine*, 222, 145–53.

77 Charles, L. E., Slaven, J. E., Mnatsakanova, A., Ma, C., Violanti, J. M., Fekedulegn, D., Andrew, M. E., Vila, B. J., and Burchfiel, C. M. (2011), 'Association of perceived stress with sleep duration and sleep quality in police officers', *International Journal of Emergency Mental Health*, 13 (4), 229–41.

78 Yang, B., Wang, Y., Cui, F., et al. (2018), 'Association between insomnia and job stress: a meta-analysis', *Sleep and Breathing*, 22 (4), 1221–31.

79 Chiang, J. J., Park, H., Almeida, D. M., Bower, J. E., Cole, S. W., Irwin, M. R., McCreath, H., Seeman, T. E., and Fuligni, A. J. (2019), 'Psychosocial stress and C-reactive protein from mid-adolescence to young adulthood', *Health Psychology: Official Journal of the Division of Health Psychology*, American Psychological Association, 38(3), 259–67.

80 Costamagna, D., Costelli, P., Sampaolesi, M., and Penna, F. (2015), 'Role of inflammation in muscle homeostasis and myogenesis', *Mediators of Inflammation*, 1–14.

81 Bodenmann, G., Atkins, D. C., Schär, M., and Poffet, V. (2010), 'The association between daily stress and sexual activity', *Journal of Family Psychology*, 24, 3, 271–9.

82 Agarwal, U., Mishra, S., Xu, J., Levin, S., Gonzales, J., and Barnard, N. (2015), 'A multicenter randomized controlled trial of a nutrition intervention program in a multiethnic adult population in the corporate setting reduces depression and anxiety and improves quality of life: the GEICO Study', *American Journal of Health Promotion*, 29 (4), 245–54.

83 Pascoe, M., Thompson, D., Jenkins, Z., and Ski, C. (2017), 'Mindfulness mediates the physiological markers of stress: systematic review and meta-analysis', *Journal of Psychiatric Research*, 95, 156–78.

84 Jackowska, M., Brown, J., Ronaldson, A., and Steptoe, A. (2015), 'The impact of a brief gratitude intervention on subjective well-being, biology and sleep', *Journal of Health Psychology*, 21 (10), 2207–17.

85 Boyd, R., and Richerson, P. (2009), 'Culture and the evolution of human cooperation', *Philosophical Transactions of the Royal Society B*, 364 (1533), 3281–8.

86 Holt-Lunstad, J., Smith, T., Layton, J., and Brayne, C. (2010), 'Social relationships and mortality risk: a meta-analytic review (social relationships and mortality)', *PLoS Medicine*, 7 (7), E1000316.

87 Valtorta, N., Kanaan, M., Gilbody, S., Ronzi, S., and Hanratty, B. (2016), 'Loneliness and social isolation as risk factors for coronary heart disease and stroke: Systematic review and meta-analysis of longitudinal observational studies', *Heart*, 102 (13), 1009–16.

88 Fox, C., Harper, A., Hyner, G., and Lyle, R. (1994), 'Loneliness, emotional repression, marital quality, and major life events in women who develop breast cancer', *Journal of Community Health*, 19 (6), 467–82.

89 Pressman, S., Cohen, S., Miller, G., Barkin, A., Rabin, B., and Treanor, J. (2005), 'Loneliness, social network size, and immune response to influenza vaccination in college freshmen', *Health Psychology*, 24 (3), 297–306.

90 Cacioppo, J., Hughes, M., Waite, L., Hawkley, L., and Thisted, R. (2006), 'Loneliness as a specific risk factor for depressive symptoms: cross-sectional and longitudinal analyses', *Psychology and Aging*, 21 (1), 140–51.

91 Teo, A., Lerrigo, R., and Rogers, M. (2013), 'The role of social isolation in social anxiety disorder: a systematic review and meta-analysis', *Journal of Anxiety Disorders*, 27 (4), 353–4.

92 Nordentoft, M., and Rubin, P. (1993), 'Mental illness and social integration among suicide attempters in Copenhagen. Comparison with the general population and a four-year follow-up study of 100 patients', *Acta Psychiatrica Scandinavica*, 88 (4), 278–85.

93 De Niro, D. A. (1995), 'Perceived alienation in individuals with residual-type schizophrenia', *Issues in Mental Health Nursing*, 16 (3), 185–200.

94 Penninkilampi, R., Casey, A., Singh, M., and Brodaty, H. (2018), 'The association between social engagement, loneliness, and risk of dementia: a systematic review and meta-analysis', *Journal of Alzheimer's Disease*, 66 (4), 1619–33.

95 Martino, J., Pegg, J., and Frates, E. (2017), 'The connection prescription: using the power of social interactions and the deep desire for connectedness to empower health and wellness', *American Journal of Lifestyle Medicine*, 11 (6), 466–75.

96 Seltzer, L. J., Prososki, A. R., Ziegler, T. E., and Pollak, S. D. (2012), 'Instant messages vs. speech: hormones and why we still need to hear each other', *Evolution and human behavior: Official Journal of the Human Behavior and Evolution Society*, 33 (1), 42–5.

97 Kiser, D., Steemers, B., Branchi, I., and Homberg, J. R. (2012), 'The reciprocal interaction between serotonin and social behaviour', *Neuroscience and Biobehavioral Reviews*, 36 (2), 786–98.

98 Jenkins, T. A., Nguyen, J. C., Polglaze, K. E., and Bertrand, P. P. (2016), 'Influence of tryptophan and serotonin on mood and cognition with a possible role of the gut–brain axis', *Nutrients*, 8 (1), 56, https://doi.org/10.3390/nu8010056.

99 Kim, E., Kubzansky, L., Soo, J., and Boehm, J. (2017), 'Maintaining healthy behavior: a prospective study of psychological well-being and physical activity', *Annals of Behavioral Medicine*, 51 (3), 337–47.

100 Sonderlund, A. L., Thilsing, T., and Sondergaard, J. (2019), 'Should social disconnectedness be included in primary-care screening for cardiometabolic disease? A systematic review of the relationship between everyday stress, social connectedness, and allostatic load', *PLoS ONE*, 14 (12), E0226717.

101 Wood, A., Rychlowska, M., Korb, S., and Niedenthal, P. (2016), 'Fashioning the face: sensorimotor simulation contributes to facial expression recognition', *Trends in Cognitive Sciences*, 20 (3), 227–40.

102 Christakis, N., and Fowler, J. (2008), 'Dynamic spread of happiness in a large social network: longitudinal analysis over 20 years in the Framingham Heart Study', *British Medical Journal*, 337 (Dec04 2), A2338.

Chapter 9: Customizing a meal plan

1 Cancello, R., Soranna, D., Brunani, A., Scacchi, M., Tagliaferri, A., Mai, S., Marzullo, P., Zambon, A., & Invitti, C. (2018), 'Analysis of predictive equations for estimating resting energy expenditure in a large cohort of morbidly obese patients', *Frontiers in Endocrinology*, 9, 367, https://doi.org/10.3389/fendo.2018.00367

2 Bosy-Westphal, A., Schautz, B., Later, W., Kehayias, J. J., Gallagher, D., and Müller, M. J. (2013), 'What makes a BIA equation unique? Validity of eight-electrode multi-frequency BIA to estimate body composition in a healthy adult population', *European Journal of Clinical Nutrition*, 67, Suppl 1, S14–S21.

3 Westerterp, K. R., Saris, W. H., van Es, M., ten Hoor, F. (1985), 'Use of the doubly labeled water technique in humans during heavy sustained exercise', *Journal of Applied Physiology*, 61 (6), 2162–7.

4 Zuromski, K., Witte, T., Smith, A., Goodwin, N., Bodell, L., Bartlett, M., and Siegfried, N. (2015), 'Increased prevalence of vegetarianism among women with eating pathology', *Eating Behaviors*, 19, 24–7.

5 Brown, A., Fuller, S., and Simic, M. (2019), 'Consensus statement on considerations for treating vegan patients with eating disorders', Royal College of Psychiatrists,

British Dietetic Association and BEAT: https://www.rcpsych.ac.uk/docs/default-source/members/faculties/eating-disorders/vegan-patients-eating-disorders-mar19.

6 Joy, E., Kussman, A., and Nattiv, A. (2016), '2016 update on eating disorders in athletes: a comprehensive narrative review with a focus on clinical assessment and management', *British Journal of Sports Medicine*, 50 (3), 154–62.

7 Beals, K. A., Brey, R. A., and Gonyou, J. B. (1999), 'Understanding the female athlete triad: eating disorders, amenorrhea, and osteoporosis', *Journal of School Health*, 69 (8), 337–40.

8 Dobner, J., and Kaser, S. (2018), 'Body mass index and the risk of infection – from underweight to obesity', *Clinical Microbiology and Infection*, 24 (1), 24–8.

9 Mintel: Food and Drink. https://www.mintel.com/press-centre/food-and-drink/brits-lose-count-of-their-calories-over-a-third-of-brits-dont-know-how-many-calories-they-consume-on-a-typical-day.

10 Centres for Disease Control and Prevention: Attempts to Lose Weight Among Adults in the United States, 2013–16, https://www.cdc.gov/nchs/products/databriefs/db313.htm.

11 Anderson, J. W., Konz, E. C., Frederich, R. C., Wood, C. L. (2001), 'Long-term weight-loss maintenance: a meta-analysis of US studies', *American Journal of Clinical Nutrition*, 74 (5), 579–84.

12 Mann, T., Tomiyama, A. J., Westling, E., Lew, A. M., Samuels, B., Chatman, J. (2007), 'Medicare's search for effective obesity treatments: diets are not the answer', *American Psychology,* 62 (3), 220–33.

13 Calton, J. B. (2010), 'Prevalence of micronutrient deficiency in popular diet plans', *Journal of the International Society of Sports Nutrition*, 7, 24.

14 Janssen, M., Busch, C., Rödiger, M., and Hamm, U. (2016), 'Motives of consumers following a vegan diet and their attitudes towards animal agriculture', *Appetite*, 105, 643–51.

15 Babio, N., Balanza, R., Basulto, J., Bulló, M., Salas-Salvadó, J. (2010), 'Dietary fibre: influence on body weight, glycemic control and plasma cholesterol profile', *Nutrición Hospitalaria*, 25, 327–40.

16 Menni, C. et al. (2017), 'Gut microbiome diversity and high-fibre intake are related to lower long-term weight gain', *International Journal of Obesity,* 41, 1099.

17 Menni, C., Jackson, M. A., Pallister, T., Steves, C. J., Spector, T. D., and Valdes, A. M. (2017), 'Gut microbiome diversity and high-fibre intake are related to lower long-term weight gain', *International Journal of Obesity*, 41 (7), 1099–1105.

18 Le Chatelier, E., Nielsen, T., Qin, J., et al. (2013), 'Richness of human gut microbiome correlates with metabolic markers', *Nature*, 500, 541–6.

19 Garthe, I., Raastad, T., Refsnes, P. E., Koivisto, A., and Sundgot-Borgen, J. (2011), 'Effect of two different weight-loss rates on body composition and strength and power-related performance in elite athletes', *International Journal of Sport Nutrition and Exercise Metabolism*, 21 (2), 97–104.

20 Chaston, T. B., Dixon, J. B., and O'Brien, P. E. (2006), 'Changes in fat-free mass during significant weight loss: a systematic review', *International Journal of Obesity*, 31 (5), 743–50.

21 Tal, A., and Wansink, B. (2013), 'Fattening fasting: hungry grocery shoppers buy more calories, not more food', *JAMA Internal Medicine*, 173 (12), 1146–8.

22 Muckelbauer, R., Sarganas, G., Grüneis, A., Müller-Nordhorn, J. (2013), 'Association between water consumption and body weight outcomes: a systematic review', *American Journal of Clinical Nutrition,* 98 (2), 282–99.

23 Slater, G. J., Dieter, B. P., Marsh, D. J., Helms, E. R., Shaw, G., and Iraki, J. (2019), 'Is an energy surplus required to maximize skeletal muscle hypertrophy associated with resistance training', *Frontiers in Nutrition*, 6, 131.

24 American College of Sports Medicine, American Dietetic Association, and Diet-itians of Canada (2000), 'Joint Position Statement: nutrition and athletic performance. American College of Sports Medicine, American Dietetic Association, and Diet-itians of Canada', *Medicine and Science in Sports and Exercise*, 32 (12), 2130–45.

Chapter 10: The recipes

1 Canuto Fernandes, D., Melo de Souza, E., and Veloso Naves, M. M. (2011), 'Soaking beans: alternative to improve nutritional value', *Semina. Ciências Biológicas e da Saúde*, 32 (2), 177–84.

ACKNOWLEDGEMENTS

To the incredible team at Penguin Random House: Connor Brown, Corinna Bolino and Alice Gordge, thank you for recognizing the need for this book, and for all your help, support, and direction throughout the process and for helping to get the message out there; to Annie Lee for all your help with scrupulous copy-editing, and everyone else working behind the scenes – you've all helped create the very best version of this book.

Thank you to my professors and colleagues at Oxford Brookes, University College London, and various other institutions, who taught me so much about the power of nutrition, alongside some skills and experiences that I'll treasure for life.

Thank you to my family and friends whose ongoing support and encouragement has always been unfaltering. To Mum and Dad, for being the best role models. To my wife Fran, for all your help and patience through some challenging times while writing this book, and to Bella, who inspires me to try and create a better future for our world. To my dear friend Max, who never got to read this book, but who I know would have been extremely proud.

A final thank you to all of my clients over the years – your dedication has been inspirational and through leading by example you have made a bigger impact on the world than you could know.

INDEX

Page references in *italics* indicate images.

Academy of Nutrition and
Dietetics 129
Adventist health studies 27–8
cancers and 33
cardiovascular disease (CVD)
and 31
dementia and 37
diabetes and 35–6
longevity and 38
magnesium and 70
potassium and 67
weight and 48–9
Alzheimer's disease
movement and 188
prevalence of, increasing 36–7
relationships and 200
sleep and 180
TMAO and 53
American College of Sports
Medicine 129, 151, 161
American Diabetes Association 49
amino acids
beta-alanine 173–6, *174*
calcium and 97
creatine and 166
HCAs and 54
iron and 77–8

meal plan and 208
protein and 118, 122–4, *123, 124,*
125, 133, 143–4
animal trials and *in vitro* studies
15, 17–18, 23–4
antibiotics *50,* 55
antioxidants 42–5, *43, 44,* 45
fibre and 62–3
iron and 80, 81
meal plan and 205, 206, 207,
208
optimizing intake 117–18
performance and 138, 140, 142,
148, 161, 173, 176
recovery and 112, 114–18
selenium and 109
supplements 45
Association for Nutrition 9
athletes 2, 3, 7, 16–17, 304
achievements of athletes who
have adopted a plant-based
diet, summary of 135–6
antioxidant supplements and 45
calcium and 92
cardiovascular disease and 29
diabetes and 36
eating disorders and 219–20